SOUNDS OF A STETHOSCOPE

An Internist's Perspective

Tanu Shweta Pandey

For my sister Dr. Shuchi Somya
The best doctor in the world

DISCLAIMER

To protect the privacy and confidentiality of patients and family members, names have been changed and minor modifications in relationships and situations have been made. As far as possible, permission was taken to share the real stories.

CONTENTS

THE TEMPEST— A VIOLENT PAIN

"Doctor, you are sick. You are sick," she says to me. She is literally yelling at me. I flinch.

"I am telling you what you tell your patients."

"Physician, heal thyself," a proverb found in the Bible, was meant to suggest examining your own shortcomings before judging others. It seemed to take on a literal meaning for me—take care of yourself before you take care of others, a sentiment undoubtedly reflected in her words and demeanor.

"Read between the lines. Listen to what I am *not* saying," she says.

I did. Cancer. The Emperor of all Maladies—the one that kills. But I am sure I don't have cancer. It must be the endometriosis. I was diagnosed fifteen years ago and had several types of treatments including laparoscopic surgery. But today I have elevated CA-125, a tumor marker for ovarian cancer.

"You need surgery," she says ominously.

I was afraid she would say that. "Can I wait a year until my son goes to college? I don't want to disturb his flow when he is a high-school junior and doing quite well."

"*No!* This needs to be done yesterday," she says.

"Well, what about my work schedule? I am completely booked in the clinic for four months and have an inpatient service coming up. Figuring out the rescheduling would be a nightmare."

"This is not an elective procedure. Do you understand me? Do you understand me?" No one has ever scolded me like this except my mother, and I feel a tear roll down my cheek.

"How do you work like this? Don't you have pain?" she asks.

Yes. Actually almost daily. Every day is a negotiation with myself. The goal is to maximize the pain control with the least amount of analgesic medications. It's Monday—no clinic, I can take the pain. Friday is long but followed by two days off—pain schmain. Tuesday and Thursday are long clinic days—I better take the ibuprofen two, maybe three times. Nights—I am good until 3:00 a.m. when the pain hits me like clockwork, waking me up. I should be up by 4:00 a.m. anyway.

"You poor child. You don't know what a normal life is." I thought I finally heard a streak of sympathy in her voice.

Normal? Normal for me is having a bottle of over-the-counter painkillers with me always. Normal for me is feeling panicky if I don't hear the rattle of the plastic container in my bag. Life has started to center around ibuprofen, Advil, Motrin, and Tylenol. I have taken eight already today, let's stop now. I should alternate between Tylenol and Advil, less toxicity to the liver and kidney. I need a metabolic panel. What if I end up in hemodialysis because of analgesic overuse like my neighbor's daughter, also a physician? Well, I took seventeen in a day once and nothing happened. I guess I got lucky. Is the generic ibuprofen as effective as the brand name? It's cheaper by a few cents. Let me buy the three-pack: I will save $1.40. Don't take *my* pain medicine; get your own.

This is new today. It has been close to two hours and it's not going away. Not fifteen, not thirty, not forty-five, not sixty minutes—two whole hours and the nagging ache is getting worse. I take two ibuprofen tablets. I hope this will not continue for the next two weeks.

It does.

It brings me to my knees. Twelve tablets of ibuprofen within three days; there has to be something different going on. A repeat in a few weeks. This is ridiculous. OK, I must find a method to deal with the pain. As soon as it starts, I will try to kill it by taking ibuprofen right away and not wait until it's severe. Take two more tablets in six hours, then take some more. Two days of this relentless swallowing of the blue-gel caps and, lo and behold, the third day is painless. So is the fourth and the rest of the two weeks. Eureka! I found a way to defeat this fiend within—crush it in the beginning, and it will not dare to appear again. Such an aha moment for me!

The surgery.

How am I going to do this? This is a horror of horrors. The General Medicine Clinic—anyone who is rescheduled in March will not get an appointment before August. What if they run out of their medications?

What about my HIV patients? I have medicine boards in six to seven weeks. I don't want to reschedule that. I have a presentation at a national conference that I will make, come hell or high water. The American College of Physicians is finally inducting me as a fellow, and I have dreamed of participating in the convocation ceremony. No, no, no. Not missing that for sure.

My projects with the residents? I must complete them before they apply for their fellowships so that they can get credit. I will have to cancel my trip to India to visit my parents. This is such bad timing.

"Trust me, you will feel so much better. I have good hands, you know."

She, my doctor, says it softly and compassionately.

I am starting to get convinced. I must speak to the boss. Let's see what she has to say. She will be so upset with me. Extra work for her. I feel the familiar niggle in my abdomen. Even minor stress can precipitate this pain. This is big. But now is not the time. Let me take two ibuprofen tablets before I speak to her. "I have bad news," I tell her. "OK," she says. "My job is to figure out who will cover for you. Your job is to get better. Take the next few days off to complete all the tests and follow up."

I feel a sensation of relief wash over me. She is something else, I am thinking. This didn't even flummox her a bit. She is like a mother. I have never felt more respect for another person than I do for her. I know in that one moment that everything will be all right.

Will it?

What if I die during the procedure? General anesthesia scares the heck out of me. I just want to live for two more years, until my son goes to college and settles in there. But what will happen to my husband? Oh well, he will find someone. My parents will be devastated, just to hear about the surgery, so I am not telling them until afterward. They are already dealing with one sick child; they do not need to worry about another.

All the thoughts are buzzing in my head simultaneously. I have to stop thinking like a drama queen. Let's take it a day at a time. I am going to watch a reality show on Bravo TV. That always makes me happy. *Shahs of Sunset* or *LA Shrinks*—they are so outside my world that I am fascinated by all that glitz, glamour, wealth, cat-fights, alcohol, vanity, and somewhat superficial life in Hollywood, Beverly Hills, and Malibu. And the thought inadvertently slips into my mind—do they have endometriosis, and how do they deal with the pain?

The surgery is impending. I am ready for it. The schedule has been taken care of. I will be OK. I know that. What I also know now is how hard it is to be a patient. To be poked, prodded, stuck, pressed in every possible way. To try to schedule and organize your life, keep all the appointments and tests, and maintain a semblance of sanity.

It's far easier to be a doctor than a patient. I would rather be the former any day.

To all physicians across the globe—heal yourself first. I did, and this book is the result of that. The surgery gave me a new life, one without pain. Every day I feel blessed to be healthy and able to make a difference. Every day I thank God that I never had to resort to taking narcotic pain-killers even once, that He saved me from becoming an addict in spite of horrendous pain, and that I can tell my story honestly and with pride.

CHAPTER 1

WHEN DREAMS COME TRUE

Toni Pruitt woke up in the middle of the night gasping for breath. She forgot to complete the task that her boss had given her. There was a deadline to meet, and now she was way past it. She jumped out of bed in panic. Her heart raced; her breathing was rapid, and her brain buzzed chaotically. She was mortified that she had missed the deadline again. She looked at the clock on her nightstand. It was 2:00 a.m. Maybe she could still finish the project before morning. Her husband was sleeping soundly. She ran up to him and shook him awake. He sat up and looked at her uncomprehendingly.

"Can you please help me? I forgot to do that task." Toni looked positively frightened as she gasped out the words.

"What task?"

"That one."

"Which one?"

"That one...the one that I was supposed to complete," she felt confused. Which task was that? Suddenly her mind went blank.

"It's OK, dear. You didn't have any task to complete. It's just a dream. Go back to sleep." He lay back and dozed off.

Feeling bewildered, Toni sat on the side of the bed and held her head in her hands, thinking hard, trying to recall the assignment that she was supposed to complete. What was it? Was this real? Was it just a dream? She was flummoxed. She started to calm down slowly and felt her breathing and heartbeat normalize. As she turned to lie down, she had an odd feeling that she never really had any incomplete task with a deadline from her boss.

This happened repeatedly, almost every night. It was the same theme—she would wake up in a panic that she had missed completing something that her boss had assigned to her at work. She experienced dread, fear, alarm, anxiety, terror, and trepidation—sometimes all at once, sometimes in moderation. Her husband and son got used to these nightly episodes and learned coping mechanisms. They would hug her gently and walk her back to her bed, speaking in soothing tones.

Toni was otherwise healthy. I had known her for a long time on a personal and professional level. She did not have any chronic diseases and did not take any prescribed medications. She had had two abdominal surgeries and a laparoscopy. She was up to date in her preventive screenings. She did not feel sad, depressed, or unhappy. The only symptom that she occasionally suffered from was insomnia. At times, it would be intractable, and at other times, she slept quite well. She could never recognize a pattern to her sleep or a temporal relation between the nightmares and insomnia, though she suspected they were both a result of stress at work.

Ironically, she really loved her job and got along well with people at work. She had achieved many of her professional goals during the past few years at her current job after going through several years of frustration and dissatisfaction with the state of her career. In fact, she thought she had her dream job. It was a good fit for her in many ways. She had what many would consider a stellar career, with many accolades and awards. She was kind, compassionate, and sensitive and considered herself a relentless advocate of social justice. She had a wonderful family life and many friends. She did not drink or smoke and indulged in many fun activities regularly. Indeed, she was living the American dream.

That's why she was confounded by her nightmares—why were they related to her job? Her dreams had come true. Were her dreams causing her nightmares? She had never experienced them prior to her current job.

The nightmares recurred for several years. When she moved to another city and changed her job, the nightmares continued on a regular basis with the same theme—just a different boss and a different work-related project. Some nights she felt less in a twilight zone. As time passed, she taught herself behavior modification techniques that helped her placate herself during an episode without getting agitated. She started feeling confident that she was getting better at dealing with her nightmares. Now she almost never disturbed her family while they were sleeping.

One night, she woke up in a frenzy that ended with her crashing through the bedroom door, diving to the floor in a heap, and getting injured. The door cracked at the point of impact and the doorjamb was grazed. The floor lamp toppled over. Toni had abrasions on her back and nicks on one knee. Her son was awake and ran from his bedroom to help her back to her bed before her husband could run up the stairs from the living room where he was working late.

It took a while for Toni to normalize that night. She had to take a pain medicine for the injury to her back. The door had to be fixed later on. Luckily, as her husband said, she did not run in the other direction toward the terrace door—she could have dived through that door and toppled over the balcony rails in her agitation, a sure-shot, fatal event from the eleventh floor of the building that they lived in. Several weeks later, her husband told her how he pulled the door blinds to the floor every night so that she could not see the door itself, a safety measure he thought would prevent her from running in that direction.

It was the last time she had a nightmare about her work and a boss; within a few days she turned in her resignation. She decided to take a sabbatical from work and focus on her health. The nightmares disappeared as if by magic. They never returned. She decided to work part-time from home with flexibility to work as many hours or days as she wanted to with no boss to terrorize her. She felt happy with her immensely improved sleep hygiene.

I believe in everything until it's disproved. So I believe in fairies, the myths, dragons. It all exists, even if it's in your mind. Who's to say that dreams and nightmares aren't as real as the here and now?

—John Lennon

Nightmares are common. Almost all of us have had at least one nightmare in our lives. It is not a pleasant experience. However, it seems a stretch to call it a disease or disorder because we don't feel sick. Sometimes we cannot even recollect what the nightmare was about. Much has been written about how to decipher our dreams and nightmares. There must be a connection with your reality, some say. I remember a close friend of mine telling me recently that she repeatedly dreams about a swamp and being sucked into it slowly, shouting for help, but not a soul is seen. She was puzzled and wondered why. In an instant, however, I could see the connection with her life. She was a highly acclaimed physician with many professional hats, including research and administrative positions; a wife to an equally successful physician; and a mother to two children, one of whom had chronic health problems. She loved to cook and had an extremely busy life that would leave anyone breathless. Yes, she was swamped every day, trying to keep up with all her commitments without any "me time" for herself, not realizing how her life had indeed become a swamp.

In this case, there was a clear-cut reflection of her reality in her subconscious self. But do all dreams and nightmares have significance? I recall having many that made absolutely no sense whatsoever—bizarre jumbles of settings and people who had no connection to one another and spoke words and sentences without any contextual background or circumstantial relation! A few were so inappropriate that I would not like to disclose them to anyone, and a few I wish someone would unravel for me, because they seemed dramatic and curiously peculiar. Furious dreamers recall being in a twilight zone, and the exact sequence of their dreams sometimes leaves them fatigued and unrested.

However, being a dreamer and having recurrent nightmares are poles apart and may have a significant clinical implication. "Nightmare disorder" has been characterized as a sleep disorder in the *Diagnostic and Statistical Manual of Mental Disorders 5*. It usually occurs during the rapid eye movement (REM) phase of sleep when all the muscles are normally relaxed and atonic—people are fast asleep in a quasi-paralyzed state. In literature, REM-related sleep behavior disorder (RBD) has been defined as the loss of the normal atonia of muscles during REM sleep, causing the subject to physically act out dreams or nightmares. These people are at the risk of acting out violent nightmares and either hurting themselves or their partners. It has been recommended that such people be evaluated as early as possible to initiate treatment, if needed, for preventing injury.

According to the *International Classification of Sleep Disorders*, specific criteria must be met for a diagnosis of RBD. Whether Toni had RBD or not, required a sleep study, polysomnography, with audiovisual recording. Treatment may consist of benzodiazepines like clonazepam that can cause daytime sedation in some people and confusion in the elderly. Melatonin improves sleep-related behavior but is a relative contraindication if the patient has depression. The Food and Drug Administration (FDA) has approved neither of these treatments because of a lack of evidence, so it is more of an expert opinion. Safety issues that need to be addressed in RBD, both for the patient and his or her partner, include safeguarding the bed and immediate surroundings.

The worrisome aspect of RBD is that at times this disorder may be a prelude to specific neurodegenerative diseases of the brain like Parkinson's disease, multiple system atrophy, and Lewy body dementia, especially if it occurs in those who are more than fifty years of age. Several published case reports describe patients with RBD who are diagnosed with degenerative diseases of the brain later in life. The REM sleep centers in the brain (like the amygdala) are the same that are affected in these diseases. Other nonspecific clinical findings that could indicate impending degenerative disease include constipation, smell problems, or mild cognitive impairment. However, it is difficult to detect a predilection based on these features or patterns because as we age, most of us experience these symptoms.

Transient RBD has also been described that is not associated with diseases of the brain and can occur during alcohol withdrawal or after use of certain medications like antidepressants. Some sleep phenomena occur during non-REM sleep, which is the phase prior to REM sleep. These include sleepwalking and other confusional states that are not considered to be a predictor of any future disorders or harmful in the long run. The sleep medicine Ambien can cause sleepwalking. This is not a sign of brain disease and disappears when the drug is discontinued. Interestingly, patients with Parkinson's disease experience frequent sleep disorders including dreams that can affect their quality of life. RBD may be one of the first symptoms that can cause a delay in the diagnosis unless the doctor has a strong suspicion. This is a good reason, therefore, to seek medical care with a specialist and proactively ask questions regarding neurological disorders if you have recurrent nightmares or vivid dreams.

An interesting finding in working women like Toni, who have frequent nightmares, is that their physiological response to nightmares can lead to depression over time. In depression, a chemical imbalance in the brain causes symptoms of sadness. Normally, the stress hormone cortisol is produced from the adrenal glands because of stimulation by the pituitary gland in the brain, which is in turn stimulated by the hypothalamus. This hypothalamic-pituitary-adrenal axis is critical to survival and response in times of stress and crisis. Normally, immediately after awakening, there is a rapid increase in the level of cortisol in the body that is thought to prepare the individual for the challenges of the day. Frequent nightmares are associated with a blunting of this response. In working women with nightmares, especially on working days, this blunting is a trait-like curious finding that causes a chemical imbalance in the brain and may be harmful over a long period by making these women prone to depressive symptoms. This is a worrisome finding.

After reading about it, I compared Toni's state of mind before and after the disappearance of her nightmares, and indeed, her mood was very different. She admitted that though she was never depressed, perhaps there was a flat affect and ongoing lack of emotional investment. She could also sense regaining her emotions after the nightmares disappeared.

Researchers have studied nightmares extensively to understand the factors that determine their occurrence. It has been proven that experiences faced during the day play a critical role in nightmares. In a Denmark study, it was concluded that nightmares occur more in blind people than those with vision. Almost a quarter of blind folks have frequent nightmares as compared to only 6 percent of sighted people. This could be explained by the fact that blind people more often experience threatening situations during the day. The fears and challenges faced by all men and women during the day thus play a critical role in the prevalence of nightmares. Work stressors, including an ornery boss, long hours, or demanding colleagues, may have been a factor in Toni's recurrent nightmares. Obviously, when these stressors were removed, her nightmares disappeared. An interesting piece of the puzzle would have been to check her cortisol level immediately after awakening—a lower cortisol level would have indicated a predilection to depression.

I have dreams, and I have had nightmares. I overcame the nightmares because of my dreams.

—Unknown

Nightmares can be strong predictors of not only depression but other psychiatric disorders as well, including a higher risk of suicide. However, currently no screening guidelines exist for primary-care physicians or sleep specialists to obtain a history of nightmares during the clinical visit. Anecdotally, such complaints may also be taken lightly and brushed aside as normal experiences of life. Like Toni, up to one-third of individuals with nightmares believe that there are no treatments for them. Open discussions with health-care providers may be vital in early treatment measures in chronic sufferers for many reasons—to suspect psychiatric problems, confirm RBD, watch out for early diagnosis of degenerative neurological disorders like Parkinson's disease, initiate treatment with medications, and prevent other complications like injuries.

Psychodynamic psychotherapy, which can help develop behavior modification strategies to combat daily routine triggers that may be the underlying cause of nightmares, is a highly regarded option for those experiencing chronic nightmares. Prazosin, an antihypertensive, has proven useful in treating nightmares linked to posttraumatic stress disorder. In a landmark study published in *JAMA* in 2001, image rehearsal therapy (IRT) is described as an effective treatment modality for victims of sexual assault and PTSD. IRT is a very simple technique in which the patient is asked to write down a nightmare, think about how to change it favorably, and paint it in in his or her mind as a mental picture. Spending a few minutes every day doing this could effectively relieve recurrence of nightmares, though it may sound too simple and almost patronizing to the victims.

For Toni, work was her stressor and a lifestyle change resulted in a quick and favorable outcome. If she experiences a recurrence, she may need a sleep study in the future, mainly to evaluate for RBD and initiate treatment. It remains to be seen if she will develop clinical evidence of a neurodegenerative disorder. Awareness of such a possibility has made her watch like a hawk for known symptoms. As an aside, she has been thankful for the respite she was able to get from the daily drudgery of work. She has found time to indulge in some of her other interests in life and found her passion in a variety of rewarding activities that she had always dreamed of. Her insomnia disappeared magically, and nightmares are a memory of the somewhat distant past. Her family is equally relieved to see the remarkable change in her overall disposition.

In a quirky way, while Toni suffered nightmares during her dream job, she was ironically able to transform her nightmares into her dreams. But she often worries about her brain and its chemical function. Her biggest concern has been about dementia since she has a strong family history. Could she suffer from dementia at an early age? What are the implications of Alzheimer's disease? How would it affect her family? Should she consider getting a living will and power of attorney? Who would make decisions for her if it happens? All these are very reasonable questions that many of my patients have asked me.

Because indeed, memories are not forever...

CHAPTER 2
MEMORIES ARE NOT FOREVER

She could remember my name
My face, our relationship,
But when her eyes fell on me,
There was a memory dip.

Sara, she said happily,
You look like Tanu today.
I wish she were here.
'Twould have made my day.

And onward she goes
Into the jumble of her mind,
An on and off switch
That's broken on rewind.

She laughs and then cries
With no whys nor wherefores,
A ship that doth sail
Further away from the shores.

After spending three days and three nights with me continuously by her bedside in a hospital room, my aunt failed to recognize me on the fourth day—just like that. She thought I was the neighbor's daughter who had come to visit her.

My uncle was sitting in a chair by her bed. For a minute, he had a quizzical look on his face, and then he corrected her. "This is Tanu. Can't you recognize her?"

"Oh, is it? I'm so sorry. I forgot." She chuckled in mortification. "I forget a lot these days."

I said nothing. I knew what was going on. I did not correct, deride, laugh at, or mock her, as many others did, including her own family members. Ten minutes later she turned toward me and asked, "Sara, how is your mother?"

"She is not Sara; she is Tanu," my uncle said with a tinge of frustration.

"My mother is doing fine, Auntie," I said. I became Sara, for that moment, to whom my aunt had always been an "auntie."

"OK, good." She lay back and fell asleep.

I stood up to smooth down her bedsheets. The sadness that engulfed me at that moment was indescribable. Here was a sixty-eight-year-old, vibrant woman, a mother and wife, who had spent her entire life in selfless devotion to her family without any desires for herself, reduced to being bedridden with progressively worsening dementia and completely dependent on others for simple activities of daily life.

Five days before, she had fallen in her living room while moving a couch. She tripped on the carpet and fell on her right hand. She suffered a complex fracture of the long bones of the forearm at the wrist, known as a Colles' fracture. This fracture frequently occurs in older postmenopausal women with weak bones, or osteoporosis. She was admitted to a local hospital in a small industrial city in India. The orthopedic specialist recommended major surgery as treatment—open reduction with internal fixation and implant. As per hospital protocol, she initially got a bed in the women's ward. Later we could choose to transfer her to a private room if we wanted to.

In the women's ward, my aunt became disoriented. The pain from the fracture and the painkillers made the underlying dementia worse, resulting in confusion and psychosis. At one point in the evening, she tried to leave the ward and "go home." She complained that the nurses were trying to rob her. The nursing staff had to hold her in the nurses' station under supervision until I made it to the hospital. I found her talking incoherently and somewhat hostile to the people around her, very unlike her usual warm self. When she saw me, she brightened up immediately. We hugged each other, and she broke down in tears and sobbed. But even in that instant, she beamed at the staff and said, "This is my niece. She is a doctor." The pride and relief in her voice was unmistakable. She had found at least one familiar face within a sea of strangers.

We moved to a private room right away. The relatively more serene surroundings and absence of strangers had a calming effect, and soon she was relaxed and restful. Her right arm was in a cast from below the elbow to the midfinger level. She waved her right arm at me and asked me why she had it. I reminded her that she'd had a fall the day before. She could not recall.

I was well aware of her slowly failing memory for the last couple of years. But I did not expect her to completely forget an injury less than twenty-four hours before that had caused a painful fracture. Little did I know that it was just the beginning.

We spent the next four days struggling with her going in and out of lucid moments and disorientation. At times, she became completely incoherent, confused, agitated, and frantic. She was calmer and more comfortable during the day, but as evening approached, her agitation became worse, a classic feature of "sundowning." Sometimes she thought she was at home and wanted to lock the doors, searched for her keys, and tried to check on her husband, who was not with us. The next night she was convinced that he had left her at home alone and checked himself into a hospital for high blood pressure. She expressed her anger at him for not letting her know and "sneaking" around. She tried repeatedly to get out of bed at night, mostly looking for her home keys. In spite of the side rails, the danger of another injury was real.

By the second day, I was convinced that any type of open surgery was going to have a poor outcome with a tumultuous postoperative recovery. After discussing the options with my family, a couple of doctor friends, and her primary orthopedic specialist, it was decided that we would proceed with closed reduction and a cast. The procedure was done under general anesthesia and went smoothly. By evening, she was starting to recover from the sedating effects of anesthesia. She ate a good meal. Family members and friends visited her, and she was able to recognize all of them. Finally, she fell asleep. By then I was exhausted too and looked forward to having a few hours of uninterrupted sleep.

Just minutes after I fell asleep, I woke up to find her hovering over me. She had managed to get out of the bed with the rails up and was trying to wake me up to go to the bathroom. I jumped out of my bed with my heart in my mouth—did she hurt herself? Fortunately, she was fine. After the trip to the bathroom, I put her back into her bed, all the while talking in gentle soothing tones with her about the risk of getting out of bed and falling. Ten minutes later, she was reaching out to the nightstand and rummaging around for her keys, mumbling incoherently. She was agitated and delirious all night long. Magically, she calmed down completely when my uncle came to visit in the morning. Within minutes, she was back to baseline, fully oriented, happy, and restful. Maybe the sunlight or maybe the sight of her partner did the trick—or both.

The whole family felt sad. We had the same thoughts—why was this happening? Is she ever going to get better? Will her memory return? Is it going to get worse? How much time does she have before she forgets everything?

None of us wants to be reminded that dementia is random, relentless, and frighteningly common.

—Laurie Graham.

Dementia is a serious disorder that must not be confused with age-related memory loss. In the latter, older people occasionally forget past as well as recent events in a patchy and sporadic manner. They usually forget pieces of events, not the entire event, and may be able to recall more later. It may or may not be associated with cognitive impairment, and almost never with psychosis or delirium. Nor does it worsen with anesthesia, drugs, or unfamiliar surroundings.

In dementia, recent memory is affected initially, whereas remote memory remains intact, and the above factors exacerbate it. Patients may be frankly psychotic at times with hallucinations and delusions that are usually associated with cognitive impairment. The memory loss is for the entire event or person, and he or she is not able to recall it later. As the disease progresses, the person may get lost, not be able to follow verbal or written directions, and lose the ability to care for others and for self.

Pathologically, simply put, there is degeneration of brain cells that results in cell death and altered chemical balance. In Alzheimer's dementia, this process is irreversible and progressive. In some of the other types, it is possible to halt the degenerative process. However, no specific treatment exists currently that can reverse the memory loss.

According to the World Health Organization, almost fifty million people suffer from dementia worldwide, with almost eight million new cases annually. This number is likely to be more than seventy-five million by 2030 and one hundred thirty-five million by 2050. More than two-thirds of these cases of dementia are because of Alzheimer's dementia. Other causes include vascular dementia related to strokes, Lewy body dementia, and frontotemporal dementia, a bunch of medical mumbo-jumbo-type names difficult to remember. In the United States, 25 percent of caregivers for adults over fifty are caring for someone with dementia, according to the Centers for Disease Control (CDC). It is the sixth-leading cause of death in the United States and almost half a million people die from Alzheimer's every year.

What factors determine who will develop dementia, especially Alzheimer's? Studies have consistently shown that multiple factors are involved, including genetics, environment, and lifestyle. However, genes merely increase the risk for developing dementia and cannot be blamed entirely for causing it. Environmental factors play a key role in the timing of the onset and rate of progression of most types of dementia.

Dementia is not a normal part of aging, contrary to what may be the current perception. It affects patients, their families, and society in many ways—physically, psychologically, economically, and socially. It can have devastating effects on people and lead to unfortunate outcomes. Who can forget the American president Ronald Reagan and his struggle with dementia? In the end, he lost his self-identity and that of the rest of the world. He even forgot that he was once Mr. President.

Reagan was the fortieth president of America from 1981 to 1989. In 1989, during a vacation trip to Mexico, he fell from a horse, resulting in a serious concussion with a subdural hematoma (bleeding in the brain) for which he underwent brain surgery. Specialists strongly believe that this unfortunate incident was momentous in the onset and rapid decline of his cognition, also known as posttraumatic dementia that occurs after a single head injury. He was formally diagnosed five years later in 1994.

Rita Hayworth, an outstanding Hollywood actor, was afflicted with it in her forties. Such an early onset is known as presenile dementia, which has a strong genetic component and an onset before the age of sixty-five. Unfortunately, she remained undiagnosed for many years in spite of fairly obvious clinical signs and symptoms. Later, she became a vibrant advocate and was depicted as the "face of Alzheimer's disease." For the past twenty-five years or so, the Alzheimer's Association has held an annual Rita Hayworth gala.

Sugar Ray Robinson, commonly cited as the best boxer of all time, was diagnosed with dementia in his sixties and passed away at sixty-seven. Repeated punches to his head during his career most likely contributed to his condition. Boxer's dementia, also known as dementia pugilistica, results from repetitive trauma to the head leading to pathological changes in the brain and degenerative encephalopathy.

Margaret Thatcher, the brilliant, former, prime minister of Britain, who was said to have died from a stroke, suffered from dementia in the last few years of her life. She had small strokes in her brain and had what is termed as vascular or multi-infarct dementia. Over a period of years, this led to changes in her brain and progressive memory loss. In a strange twist of fate, history has noted her strong bonds with Ronald Reagan. In 2004, though she was physically present at his funeral, her eulogy was delivered via a prerecorded message broadcast on television screens. It was deemed that her mental status, compromised because of dementia, would not allow her to speak live. Two formidable leaders of the strongest countries in the world—powerful political juggernauts and once brilliant minds—were reduced to nothing by the same devastating illness, albeit of entirely different causes.

With the advancement of medicine and research, it is now possible to evaluate speech patterns and predict the risk for dementia. In the case of Reagan, several studies on his speech early in his presidency were described after his death as red flags that could have predicted his future illness because of his use of repetition and vague terminology. Mild forms of dementia, including AD, are associated with biochemical changes in the cerebrospinal fluid in the brain that are markers of neural dysfunction. The upside of such technology is that it makes possible early diagnosis and possible treatment that may halt the progress of dementia. At least the underlying causes can surely be addressed, like trauma, strokes, and so on.

At some point, there would simply be no point.

—Lisa Genova, *Still Alice*

As dementia progresses to an advanced stage, the patient may have poor nutritional intake resulting in dehydration and illnesses like pneumonia and urinary tract infections. In such cases, it is best to avoid gastric tubes to feed the patient and instead maintain hydration via parenteral means like intravenous fluids and fully assisted comfort feeding. At this stage, symptom management becomes fundamental. Pain control, mouth hygiene, suction of fluids, sedation, and oxygen therapy may be needed. Narcotics like morphine are often useful in controlling pain, as well as inducing relaxation. Most often, such advanced patients may get a lower respiratory tract infection or pneumonia, which may be the reason for death. Avoiding aspiration of saliva and other fluids or food by keeping the patient upright with the bed end elevated can avoid pneumonia in many cases. Antibiotics for infections fall in the gray zone—should we prescribe them or not? Patient care includes individualized shared decision making among families, primary physicians, and palliative care specialists.

End-of-life issues in dementia are critical. Recognizing dementia as a terminal disease by the physicians and families is the first step toward avoiding complexities in the overall situation related to expectations and goals of care. Educating the family about the prognosis and options for palliative care is vital. Addressing legal issues like a power of attorney to make medical decisions and advanced directives with a living will make it more manageable for the family.

Ethics play a tremendously meaningful role in caring for a patient with dementia. In developing countries with poor resources, there is an inherent concept of home hospice-type care for the terminally ill. Most patients die at home, among their loved ones, in the comfort of their familiar surroundings. It is a kind and compassionate practice in some ways. However, palliative care as a specialty is not practiced widely, and there is a huge deficit in awareness, even within the medical community, about empathic care for the elderly. Narcotic pain medication is strictly prohibited and difficult to provide. The concept of medically supervised comfort care is poorly established. Often, this results in the painful and excruciating ebbing of life over extended periods. Mother Teresa, well known for her charitable work for the terminally ill, could provide only aspirin to patients in her camps, in spite of the presence of advanced cancer with intractable pain syndromes.

In the West, however, hospice is a choice, an option that the family members have, to keep one of their own in comfort and allow him or her to die in peace. Innumerable times over years of practice, I have struggled with families who fail to understand the concept of hospice for advanced dementia patients. Recently, the family of a ninety-nine-year-old mother of four kept her alive in the hospital with strict instructions not to administer morphine or other sedating agents. Her primary caregiver, her second daughter, had unrealistic expectations that she would be able to take her home. No amount of frank discussion could convince her otherwise. I watched sorrowfully as her mother's life ebbed slowly and painfully away under our eyes until she took her last breath more than forty hours later. A harsh and cruel choice that could have easily been made much more humane and considerate. It reminded me of a quote that I had read somewhere: death may indeed be a kinder option than the harsh callousness of dementia.

Such experiences also made me aware of how difficult it can be for family members to let go of a loved one. It can create friction among siblings with differing opinions and underlying tension beget by the multiple psychosocial and legal issues that arise. It can break apart families and take away a lot more than what families bargained for, especially in the absence of a living will. A long time ago, I had to call emergency services to transfer a ninety-year-old woman with dementia from my clinic to the ER after she claimed to have had suicidal thoughts repeatedly with plans to use a gun. She lived with her daughter and son-in-law in a house that belonged to her. In the hospital, social workers arranged for long-term care at a nursing home after she was deemed clinically unfit to care for herself. This led to authorities auctioning her house to pay for her care and resulted in the automatic eviction of her daughter and son-in-law. I felt guilty about this outcome, but there was no other option. If only my patient had completed a living will with her daughter as the heir of her house, this could have been avoided.

Julianne Moore won multiple awards, including an Oscar in 2014, for her portrayal of a Columbia University linguistics professor with early onset of Alzheimer's in the movie "Still Alice," based on a bestseller of the same name. The film was applauded for its sensitive portrayal of a deadly disorder in a poignant manner that highlighted the long-lasting ripples of dementia experienced by close family members. On a personal level, it seemed to touch a nerve with me. I have watched my family members deal with my aunt, whose children live far away. They sometimes spend hours on FaceTime and the phone with no hope of improvement in spite of multiple medications. I know that the end is near and that it is not going to be pretty. Indeed, it's heartbreaking to even remotely acknowledge this fact.

For me, as the only physician in the family, the most difficult part has been trying to explain the truth honestly to everyone. I am trying to prepare them for what is coming, to help the children cope with losing the person they knew as their mother, and to sort their feelings of frustration with her often chaotic and frenzied disposition. I try to persuade them not to lose patience at her obsession with a single topic day after day, and I try to help them understand a little more profoundly the many perplexing pieces that make this puzzle. As laypersons, they are bewildered by her randomness, disconcerted by her memory loss, and incredibly anxious about her fretful behavior. I fear that what I may be witnessing is a prelude to family burnout in the future. Sadly, I see no way to prevent it or even delay it.

Someone rightly said that there are never any survivors of dementia. We as a society must address this problem sooner rather than later. The inherent issues are the same everywhere—care for the elderly is unique in its needs and demands a cohesive treatment plan among several specialties like geriatrics, internal medicine, palliative care, and so on. Many of these specialties are not available to medical students in the developing world. The medical disorders are the same. Most of the medical books are also the same. The training is diverse, driven by cultural roots and mindset. This makes the practice of medicine dissimilar in different parts of the world. In the West, technology and state-of-the-art equipment blend with evidence-based guidelines, whereas in the East, affordability of and accessibility to medical care are the primary issues. And the outcomes? Good and bad outcomes are witnessed on both sides of the world in roughly equal measures. In spite of generalizations and stereotypes, it would be incorrect to say that the outcome of medical care is necessarily better in the Western world.

Though comparisons are odious, my personal experiences make it easy for me to examine, describe, and compare notes between the country I grew up in (a third-world country) and the one that I currently live and work in (a superpower). Is one better than the other based on outcomes?

CHAPTER 3
NOTES FROM THE
THIRD WORLD

A Short History of Medicine
2000 BC—"Here, eat this root."
1000 BC—"That root is heathen. Say this prayer."
AD 1850—"That prayer is superstition. Drink this potion."
AD 1940—"That potion is snake oil. Swallow this pill."
AD 1985—"That pill is ineffective. Take this antibiotic."
AD 2000—"That antibiotic is artificial. Here, eat this root."

—Author Unknown

The circle is complete. The science of medicine is black and white, as described in the medical books. The art of medicine, on the other hand, is far more complex. Often, the two are divergent precepts. As I sat in my father's hospital room in New Delhi, India, waiting for his turn to be taken to surgery one morning, I had the time to reflect on what exactly constitutes medical care: guideline driven, on-demand care as in the United States; guideline-driven, socialized medicine as in Canada and Britain; "point of care" practice as in the developing countries; or just commonsense, no-harm-done, cost-effective care that is the fundamental core of the Hippocratic oath that all physicians commit to at the start of their careers.

Is one way better than the other? Does it matter how we practice medicine as long as the outcome is good for the patient?

My recent experiences in India with three close associates who were sick and did not have health-insurance coverage (as is usual) has forced me to rethink the key concepts of health-care delivery:

- Early clinical diagnosis and treatment are the most critical elements for quick recovery irrespective of modern-day investigative technology and guidelines.
- Treatment options must be individualized based on the patient profile.
- Contemporary, expensive, state-of-the-art care is not the monopoly of developed nations and can be available anywhere for a price.

Diagnosis is not the end, but the beginning of practice.

—Martin H. Fischer

The first critical sickness developed acutely in a close friend in a small, overcrowded township in India. There was a sudden onset of low-grade fever with malaise, fatigue, and an occasional slight cough without dyspnea or chest pain. The elderly grandmother insisted that the fever appeared only in the afternoon every day. She lived in a small town that was primarily tribal and considered one of the most backward areas of the country, though the burgeoning middle class had a contemporary mind-set about education, progress, technology, and gender equality. I grew up and received my entire education in that town, including medical school. Medicines were freely available over the counter, even antibiotics, and some controlled substances. Self-medication was common, and my friend empirically treated herself with amoxicillin initially—a standard local practice, based on the assumption that it would resolve any infection that was causing the fever. It was also very cheap; for less than a dollar, we can buy a weeklong antibiotic dose.

After four days passed without a response to amoxicillin, I suggested that she consult another friend and medical-school classmate, a renowned doctor in the city. Within the next few hours, an outpatient X-ray of the chest revealed that the right lung was collapsed because of excessive fluid collection in the outer linings, medically known as "massive pleural effusion," with near complete opacification of the right lung field. It is most commonly seen when an infection in the lungs causes inflammation and oozing of abnormal fluid from the cells lining the lung membranes, for example in pneumonia. The doctor's empirical diagnosis, however, was not pneumonia but tuberculosis, and he initiated antituberculous treatment immediately while awaiting the result of the skin test for tuberculosis. Within three days, she improved dramatically with resolution of fever and a week later was almost back to normal.

As a physician practicing in America, I reacted with near panic when I saw the chest X-ray and anticipated a hospital admission, complex procedures like diagnostic and therapeutic thoracentesis (removal of the fluid from the lungs with large bore needles for symptom relief and testing for infection, cancer, etc.), complications from questionable procedural skills of physicians, possible alternative diagnoses, and so on. I spoke to my doctor friend extensively, and he reassured me that she did not need any more tests. Twelve days after the treatment began, a follow-up, chest X-ray revealed near complete disappearance of the fluid collection and reversal of the lung collapse without any underlying residual infection. Six months later, she had recovered completely. The entire treatment cost less than $300.

A very sick patient was effectively managed for a serious illness purely utilizing strong clinical skills in an outpatient setting, without any invasive procedures, costly diagnostic tests, hospital admission, or unnecessary delay in treatment initiation.

*It is much more important to know what sort of a patient
has disease than what sort of disease a patient has.*

—Sir William Osler

A few days later, I received a call that my aunt had fractured her wrist after a fall, the same aunt described in the previous chapter. She was sixty-eight years old and had progressive moderately advanced Alzheimer's dementia. While trying to arrange the sofa in the living room, she tripped on the carpet. She had a long-standing, movement disorder that had affected her muscle and limb coordination significantly. Her bones were thinned out because of osteoporosis from lack of the female hormone, estrogen that is seen in all postmenopausal women. Additionally, she was on a medication for seizures that had likely aggravated the osteoporosis as a side effect. She tried to break her fall with her outstretched hand and the weight of her whole body was too much for the frail bones. As expected, X-rays revealed a complex forearm bone fracture, called a Colle's fracture, which is commonly seen in postmenopausal women who have osteoporosis. My mother and maternal grandmother also had this fracture.

She was admitted at a local hospital where surgical treatment with an expensive, implant placement was recommended. The steel company that employed my uncle before his retirement ran the hospital. I was impressed that such expertise was available at a small-city institution that was obviously well run. The conventional nonsurgical option (closed reduction and cast application) was not even discussed as an alternative, and preoperative medical clearance was initiated prior to the surgery.

As her primary caregiver at that time, I had to make the critical decision on her behalf in conjunction with her children and husband. When she became agitated and confused because of dementia within the unfamiliar confines of the hospital, I knew that the surgical procedure would be a disaster postoperatively owing to her unstable mental status. Implant infection and rejection would be a grave complication that could quickly proceed to excessive morbidity with a prolonged hospital stay and even death.

I discussed my concerns with the surgeon and suggested that we should opt for the more conservative procedure—realignment of bones and cast without surgery or implant. The surgeon was hesitant to proceed with this option since the complexity of the fracture would inevitably result in healing with deformity of the hand, residual pain in the wrist, and delayed functional recovery. He cited clinical guidelines and the latest research. My argument was that with advanced dementia, a smooth recovery would be impossible after a complex surgery, whereas she could live with deformity and mild pain. It was time to make the final decision. The surgeon was rightly cautious about making decisions with a family member who was unrelated to the patient. He suggested that I let her husband and children decide, as "we could all get into trouble."

Of course I agreed with him and was in constant communication with them. They agreed to proceed with the conservative option.

To be completely sure, we consulted by phone with a senior orthopedic surgeon in Chicago, who was also a family friend, as well as another doctor in New Delhi. Both of them agreed that going conservative was the best option. My aunt has since then recovered smoothly and without unexpected complications, other than the slightly crooked wrist, which was expected. The entire treatment cost less than $500.

An elderly woman with dementia was effectively treated with conservative management for a fracture, though state-of-the-art, modern surgical expertise was available at low cost. The case exemplifies the rule that each patient deserves treatment customized to his or her individual needs in spite of the availability of cutting-edge, medical technology and equipment.

If you are too smart to pay the doctor,
you had better be too smart to get ill.

—African Proverb

My seventy-seven-year-old father had been suffering from hemorrhoids for several years. The condition is commonly known as piles and occurs because of enlargement of the veins in the rectum, resulting in bleeding through the anus, sometimes with bowel movements, and sometimes spontaneously. Bleeding can be minimal with just spotting or torrential with potential exsanguination. Since it is venous blood, it can be challenging to stop the bleeding by pressure alone or other conservative measures. As the veins grow larger because of pressure from gravity or during bowel straining, there can be a protrusion of the veins out of the anus. This necessitates manually pushing the veins back in for comfort after every bowel movement or with abdominal straining, and it puts the patient at high risk for infection and excessive bleeding, both serious complications.

In the last six months, my father had progressive worsening of symptoms with prolapse of the hemorrhoids and poor quality of life. He had several investigative procedures done, including proctoscopy, flexible sigmoidoscopy, and colonoscopy. The final recommendation from the gastroenterologist was urgent hemorrhoid surgery if complications were to be prevented. Surgical options were either traditional excision (cutting out the veins) or a new, state-of-the-art, stapling procedure, also known as a procedure for prolapse and hemorrhoids (PPH).

The small town where he lived had expert surgeons, competent in conventional excision. The procedure was associated with a very painful postoperative recovery, which was a strong deterrent to him, and he refused to undergo this procedure. On the other hand, there were several advantages to stapling: the postoperative recovery was quicker, it was much less painful, and it was generally well tolerated with early discharge from the hospital. However, this required an expensive instrument (the stapler), which was only available in the big cities and tertiary care centers and should be performed by a surgeon with known expertise in minimally invasive surgery.

This procedure was not available in the city where my father lived. I would have to fly my father to New Delhi to a state-of-the-art private hospital well known in South Asia for its international clientele and spend at least one week there, a daunting prospect for me with safety concerns, fear of the unknown, and a potential logistics nightmare. Regardless of expected difficulties, I was able to convince my father to agree to the treatment. The trip was uneventful, and the surgery was free of complications. He is now doing well and is very happy about the outcome. The entire treatment cost $3,500. If he had opted for the traditional surgery in his hometown, the cost would have been less than $500.

My father was able to get a relatively minor surgery at seven times the cost of a traditional procedure with a quick recovery and discharge at a fancy "five-star" institution, inherently because we could afford it.

Medicine is a science of uncertainty and an art of probability.

—Sir William Osler

Three patients, three disorders, three cities, three provider teams, three different price tags, one outcome—good. In none of the cases was overall medical management directed by any existing international clinical guidelines. Let us imagine what would have happened if they lived in the United States.

First, my friend with tuberculosis would go to the emergency room. After the chest X-ray, she would be admitted to a hospital under a primary-care physician or hospitalist. A pulmonologist (lung specialist) would be consulted and would perform a thoracentesis procedure to drain the fluid from the right lung. The fluid would be sent for expensive tests including culture for bacterial organisms, sensitivity to antibiotics, cytology for cancer, and so on. In all probability, a CT scan of the chest would be done, exposing her to radiation and intravenous contrast dye, both of which are harmful. Tuberculosis medicines would not be initiated immediately. Instead, several rounds of antibiotics, possibly intravenous, would be prescribed. The total bill would be approximately $15,000 or more, some of which may be covered by health-insurance plans if she were enrolled in one.

My aunt's situation would be different too. After admission to a hospital under a primary-care physician or hospitalist, an orthopedic surgeon would be consulted for the fracture, a neurologist for dementia and seizures, a psychiatrist for psychosis, and social services for a home-safety evaluation. There would be a discussion about brief (possibly three-week) nursing-home stay after hospital discharge for physical therapy and recovery from her altered mental status. The surgical options would be the same but insurance coverage would be the deciding factor instead of the most appropriate procedure for her. The total bill could be anywhere from $20,000 to $25,000 or even more.

As far as my father is concerned, his care was the most comparable to medical care in the West. Some things would be better and some worse. The surgery would be an outpatient day procedure instead of a three-day, hospital admission. Insurance coverage would be critical in opting for the procedure of personal choice—newer treatments are often not covered by most health-insurance plans and stapling may not be considered as the most cost-effective choice. The choice of a surgeon for an elective surgery would also be an in-network doctor, perhaps without an option to choose an internationally renowned surgeon in a faraway city out of state. The cost could be anywhere between $10,000 and $25,000.

The art of medicine consists of amusing the patient while nature cures the disease.

—*Voltaire*

"Evidence-based medicine" is defined as the use of current, scientific-research evidence in medicine for making decisions for patient care. These clinical guidelines are often based on the results from randomized clinical trials, considered the holy grail in medical research, albeit an expensive one. It is conventionally considered the best way to practice medicine because it standardizes care. However, it is a fact that medical care in developing countries lacks evidence-based guidelines and cost-effective, public policies. Expensive research is impossible because of a lack of adequate resources. The concept of population-based public health is not as established as in the Western world. Heterogeneity is the norm and quality-of-care benchmarks are almost nonexistent. Some would say that care is undeniably better in the United States than in India. I wouldn't disagree with them. But my experiences in India left me wondering about what really constitutes good medical care.

Is evidence-based practice the best type of practice?

"Standard of care" and "best practice" are terms that are broadly used to indicate what most reasonably qualified providers or institutions do in a similar clinical scenario. Such practices may not have the backing of robust scientific data grounded on clinical trials, but they still find a place in day-to-day practice in western countries. The fact is that when research is not possible or has not been done for any reason, best practices are established that lead to good outcomes. In countries like India, research is scant and Western scientific data that is applicable to a predominantly Caucasian population may not be valid. Thus, best practices are very popular. These integrate the clinical expertise of the provider based on experience. In the case of my friend with tuberculosis, the physician had established that anyone living in the area of his practice with those particular symptoms, signs, and radiological evidence had tuberculosis unless proven otherwise. He wasted no time in prescribing treatment immediately, even though I secretly balked at it, having become quite "Americanized" in my medical assessment.

So why do we spend so much of our time learning about guidelines for diseases? As an educator for medical students, residents, and fellows, I have invariably underscored the importance of not just learning the components of clinical guidelines but also interpreting the research behind them. Only a fraction of what we practice is based on evidence that is derived from randomized clinical trials, arguably considered the best kind of research. The rest is an assortment of weaker research models, expert opinions, observational data, and subjective judgment. Sometimes these guidelines are reverted. We must use guidelines to do what they are meant for—to guide us in clinical care. It is an irrefutable fact that doctors spend a sizeable part of their time trying to save lives in emergent, urgent, and demanding situations where guidelines literally go for a toss. We do what we have to do to save a life. Often this means thinking out of the box and improvising our care within the resources available. I daresay this kind of medical care is the norm in third-world countries and saves millions of lives routinely.

In defense of clinical guidelines, their meager existence in developing countries can result in haphazard and fragmented care. Patients are vulnerable to paternalistic decision making at the hands of health-care providers and can get swindled financially. An absence of regulatory policies makes it worse. Fortunately, I was able to make decisions for my associates that were suitable for them. Not everyone has the same access to care that we did, and lack of basic infrastructure, rather than physician expertise, is a critical problem. Strengthening the health system as a whole with improving access to cost-effective, evidence-based, culturally appropriate care remains an overwhelming task and a critical element of the agenda for not just the governing bodies but also for international peer institutions like the World Health Organization.

"Cultural competence in medicine," another frequently addressed concept in the United States, was evident in my aunt's care. Delivery of care based on understanding the local cultural diversity and inherent beliefs is now considered a critical component of patient-centered care. There was concern from the medical team that the decisions were being made by a distant relative, not the next of kin, an appropriate response in this case. Even though I knew that the whole family looked to me for making decisions on their behalf, I still went ahead and ensured that the opinions of my uncle and their children (who were not there) were conveyed to the operating surgeon.

The broad underlying principle of cultural competence in medicine is that interactions aimed at individualizing health care rather than standardizing it, results in improvement in quality of care. It seems to be at odds with evidence-based medicine, which primarily aims for standardizing care with guidelines, not individualizing it. Critics of guideline-based care have cited problems related to lack of adherence by practitioners. Stereotyping clinical care in a one-dimensional framework can be fraught with poor outcomes without integrating cultural, ethnic, and personal health beliefs.

In the case of my father, the care that he was able to receive was directly related to affordability. We could choose the best doctors, multiple specialist opinions, a fancy hospital, a luxury private suite in the hospital, optimal travel modes, and ideal postoperative care. He strongly believed he would be better off with stapling than excision, and his wishes were fulfilled even though it was more expensive—a strong example of cultural competence in medicine.

It may seem that cultural competence is just a cog in the "third-world wheel"—that it has little, if any, implications in settings in the Western world. However, the term itself originated in the United States, a country steeped in ethnic diversity and multicultural traditions. There are innumerable instances of medical care that had to be tweaked creatively to be in harmony with the patient's personal beliefs and values. The best example of such a faith-based ingenuity is how we take care of Jehovah's Witnesses, members of a sect of Christianity with unique principles that can create significant challenges for health-care providers. Yet, we have found incredible ways to face these encounters without compromising the result. The core principle of practicing medicine is that what works for one patient may not work for another—good drug/bad drug, good surgery/bad surgery, good test/bad test, good blood/bad blood...

CHAPTER 4
GOOD BLOOD/BAD BLOOD

Barbara Smith (name changed) was tired. She had been tired for a long time. She had little energy for activities of daily life. She could hardly walk up the stairs to go to her bedroom. She fell asleep several times a day. Occasionally she felt breathless after walking short distances. This had been going on for a while without her realizing what a toll it was taking on her.

One day, she felt pressure under her left breast while cleaning her bathroom.

It came suddenly and took her completely by surprise. She had never experienced this before. It was a dull ache, a soreness in her chest, like a fist thump. She ignored it for a few minutes and continued with her cleaning. When the pain did not go away, she decided to rest for a few minutes. She dropped the mop and settled down on a recliner in front of the TV. She felt the discomfort subside. Curious to understand why she was hurting, she poked her chest with her fingers. There was no tenderness.

"Ah, well! Let's get back to what I was doing. Gotta move fast," she thought.

She walked into the bathroom and bent down to pick up the mop. Slightly breathless, she plopped the mop into the bathtub and went back and forth with it for a few minutes. The tap was a little rusted, and she would have to take care of that later.

There it was again. The pressure. This time, much more intense. Like someone was sitting on her chest. Barbara stood transfixed, too frightened to move. She laid the mop down gently and put her hand to her chest.

"This can't be good," she thought.

"Am I having a heart attack? From scrubbing the bathtub?" She felt perplexed.

She walked slowly to her living room and reached for the phone. She dialed 911. The paramedics brought her to the emergency room of my hospital, and that is where I met her for the first time.

At ERs across the country, chest pain is triaged as an acute emergency, anticipating an ongoing heart attack, for which "time is muscle"—the earlier we diagnose it, the quicker we can start treatment and save heart muscle from dying because of a lack of blood supply and oxygen.

Barbara did not have a heart attack. On the other hand, tests revealed that she was anemic with a hemoglobin level of four grams (the normal range is 12–14 grams). Hemoglobin is the iron-laden protein in the red blood cells that transports oxygen to the tissues. The low level caused a shortage of oxygen supply to the heart muscles and caused them to start dying, known as muscle necrosis in "medicalese," resulting in the chest pain. This was tantamount to an inadvertent stress test for the heart. The principle is the same as running on the treadmill to test the blood flow to the coronaries. When the heart is stressed (either by treadmill use, physical exertion, or because of anemia), the demand for oxygen is higher than the supply.

However, Barbara had angina rather than a myocardial infarction, since her heart muscles did not completely die. All her symptoms of fatigue, shortness of breath, and sleepiness made sense—the anemia was responsible for them. Since angina is a symptom of coronary artery disease, the anemia had unmasked an underlying thickening of her arteries in the heart, probably because of plaque formation and/or calcification. Getting her hemoglobin up to normal would resolve all these symptoms; we would have to address the coronary disease separately. Barbara faced two critical issues: first, to find out why she was anemic and second, to determine how we could treat it to elevate the hemoglobin level to normal. The first issue involved performing other tests for measuring iron, vitamin B12, and folic acid levels—the deficiencies of which can cause anemia—and doing procedures like upper endoscopy and colonoscopy to evaluate for a bleeding site in the gastrointestinal tract.

The second issue seemed pretty straightforward to treat—add oral iron, B12, or folic acid supplements if the levels were low and consider blood transfusion as soon as possible since she had anginal chest pain and was at increased risk for a heart attack. There is substantial scientific evidence that the risk of death increases with hemoglobin levels below five grams. The goal of transfusion would be to keep the hemoglobin at eight grams or higher. She would need two to three units of packed red-cell transfusion for this. This would offset the lack of adequate oxygen supply to the heart muscle right away.

But there was a problem. It was not as simple as it looked.

Barbara was a Jehovah's Witness. Adherents of this faith are forbidden to accept a transfusion of blood and its products, an action that could revoke their membership in their church and trigger instructions for other Jehovah's Witness followers to shun them. This is a scenario that is encountered by almost all medical professionals in the United States (and perhaps globally) at some point in their career. The premise remains the same—a patient needs transfusions of whole blood or its four products (red cell, white cell, platelets, and plasma) but cannot receive them because of his or her faith. It leaves us in a quandary—what do we do, especially when it could be lifesaving? What if advanced directives to never transfuse are not available? What happens in an emergency situation? Are children treated differently? It becomes important to understand the various aspects of the Jehovah's Witness faith and be prepared to deal with this situation in the most logical, ethical, and sensitive way possible.

The Jehovah's Witness society is a fundamental Christian sect that has certain beliefs that are unique to that religion. Adherents do not enroll in the national armed forces or salute the flag. They do not celebrate birthdays or show political allegiance. They follow the Bible as the true word of God and do not celebrate Christmas. In 1945, the Watch Tower Bible and Tract Society, which is the legislating body of the Jehovah's Witnesses, interpreted certain scripts from the Bible as prohibiting blood in any form from another person. Accepting blood transfusions from other human beings is considered equivalent to "eating blood," Since then, Jehovah's

Witnesses clearly indicate that transfusion of blood or its products is not acceptable. The sin scale of accepting a transfusion is as high as immoral-sexual behavior.

We encounter all four fundamental principles of ethics in this setting. There's *autonomy*—the right of the patient to make a decision that we must respect which in this case is refusing a blood transfusion. Then there is *beneficence*—the moral principle of doing good, which in this case is the health-care providers promoting what is best for the patient that is transfusing blood. *Nonmaleficence*, or do not harm, is explicit in the doctor's decision—do the benefits outweigh the harms from transfusion? No transfusion can be given without the patient's consent. As for *justice*, there are more than a few queries. Is the patient's decision fair? Is the doctor's decision fair? Are we providing equality of care to such patients? Is it reasonable to disqualify or bar a Jehovah's Witness patient from church if he or she decides to accept a lifesaving transfusion?

Such patients present an exceptional challenge to health-care providers when they need transfusions of blood products—for example, after major surgery or trauma—both associated with blood loss. Alternate ways to compensate for these requirements must be considered to honor and respect the beliefs of Jehovah's Witnesses. Guidelines have been published to assist doctors in minimizing blood loss during procedures and options to be considered when anticipating such loss. Minimally invasive surgery is preferred when possible, and surgeons are advised to take extra care to prevent oozing or minor bleeding from the surgical site. Occasionally, purposely lowering the blood pressure and/or temperature during anesthesia may be practiced to lower the chances of bleeding. A whole new specialty of "bloodless medicine" has sprung up in many medical centers.

In the year 2000, in what is considered a momentous change of position, the Watch Tower declared that administration of certain fractions of blood would depend on the personal choice of each follower and such actions would not be reason enough for ostracism. This was a welcome decision that altered the possibilities for Jehovah's Witness patients substantially. There are certain synthetic products and minor blood fragments that can now be transfused if indicated. These include intravenous albumin, synthetic colloids, clotting factors (like recombinant Factor VIIa used in hemophilia and occasionally in trauma patients with bleeding complications), immunoglobulins, iron transfusion, and erythropoietin (a synthetic hormone given as injections to boost red-cell production). Procedures like hemodialysis and cardiopulmonary bypass are acceptable. In patients with anemia like Barbara, who need major surgery, iron transfusions and erythropoietin injections prior to the procedure can increase the hemoglobin levels to some degree but need time, often several weeks, to show results.

Autologous predonation—patients donating blood to themselves prior to a surgical procedure, a critical solution to prepare for surgeries that incur blood loss and may need to be replenished for better healing and early recovery—is not acceptable to Jehovah's Witnesses. Isovolemic hemodilution, on the other hand, is appropriate when needed and does not conflict with the faith. It is a volume-management technique in which blood from the patient is collected *during* the surgical procedure postanesthesia, to be used if needed in the perioperative period. At the same time as the blood collection, intravascular volume is maintained by a concurrent intravenous transfusion of crystalloid or colloid solution. Jehovah's Witness patients find this acceptable as long as a continuous circuit with the patient's system is maintained at all times. Other more complex alternatives like hypervolemic hemodilution, intra- and postoperative cell salvage, and red-blood-cell substitutes, are not widely available and may be an option at the discretion of the patient.

As far as Jehovah's Witness children and pregnant women are concerned, the facts are somewhat gray. The parental right to make decisions on behalf of their children or unborn fetus is widely respected by health-care providers. However, if such decisions can harm or permanently impair children, then it becomes controversial. Allowing a child to die because of the lack of a blood transfusion makes the doctor vulnerable to prosecution, whereas transfusing blood products against a religious belief can be considered assault. Parents have a say in this matter but rules are different across the world. In Britain, children below sixteen years of age may be able to give consent for a transfusion if they understand the benefits and risks of doing so in the context of their illness. Other countries, like Canada, do not support the notion that adolescents have the maturity to make serious medical decisions like this. The position of the American Academy of Pediatrics is to respect religious beliefs and avoid conflict. However, the health of the child is paramount, though inconsistent legal opinions abound in the United States. At times, when an elective surgery cannot be performed without a blood transfusion, a court order has been sought that allows transfusion as a lifesaving measure. In emergency cases, when there is no time for a court order, transfusions may be given to save the child. In Australia, the health of the child is more important than the consent of the parent for transfusion as a lifesaving measure. The literature is replete with descriptions of many cases in the legal system that involve children of Jehovah's Witness parents. The common thread is that parental rights exist but do not extend to life-and-death authority over children.

There are also instances of dissident Jehovah's Witness followers who do not fully agree with this aspect of their faith. Theoretically, a Jehovah's Witness patient may choose to receive a blood transfusion and not confess to his or her congregation. Patient confidentiality on the part of the medical team would prohibit this information from being shared with anyone other than who the patient chooses. That this happens in reality is a moot point, with no way of really knowing without breaking the laws of privacy and confidentiality.

In my thirty years in medicine, I have never witnessed a Jehovah's Witness patient die following refusal of a transfusion. Honestly, I am not sure what would be ethically and legally the best way to act in such a situation when death is imminent. I know of a sixty-year-old man who had myelodysplastic syndrome with leukemia and chose not to get transfusions that would have elevated his hemoglobin to a safe level where he could be eligible for other treatments like new chemotherapy or stem-cell treatment. He held on to his faith in total devotion and proclaimed that he was nothing without it. The entire medical team, his family, and friends supported him in his choices. Eventually he passed away from complications of the disease, fully aware that he could have perhaps lived longer with these treatments. There was no question of transfusions to save his life. Thus, as far as possible, respecting religious beliefs of patients is vital and fundamental as long as the patient is competent and understands the outcomes. For Barbara, that is exactly what we did since she had a higher risk of heart attack but not impending death. She was found to have very low levels of iron, which we replenished with iron transfusions. She received erythropoietin injections to stimulate red-cell production. She had close monitoring after discharge and experienced a gradual rise of the hemoglobin level in the following weeks. Further tests revealed a bacterial infection in her stomach that had caused an ulcer formation. Over time, she exuded tiny amounts of blood from this ulcer which was the cause of anemia. The infection was treated with antibiotics, and medications to heal the ulcer were prescribed. Once her hemoglobin level was normalized, she never experienced chest pain again. A cardiology consultation was solicited, and the protocol for heart disease was followed, though aspirin or any other blood thinner was not prescribed immediately because of the ulcer.

Overall, this was a straightforward case that had a good outcome with a holistic approach. It makes me think about patients who are not Jehovah's Witnesses—are we too quick to transfuse blood products when it's not quite necessary? If Barbara were not a Jehovah's Witness, what would have we done?

In all likelihood, she would have received one or two units of blood. Health-care providers have long been known to use blood transfusions liberally. Early on in my career as a medical student and resident, I witnessed senior physicians transfusing at the slightest hint of anemia because they wanted to keep the level of hemoglobin above eight grams, an arbitrary value that was as random as the pain scale or the degree of edema (swelling) of the leg. As I grew up, I realized that nothing in medicine is black and white—shades of gray number more than just fifty. A level of eight is just that, a number without any clinical relevance that can be defined by meaningful outcomes, a number that eases the medical team for unknown reasons, a number to check off our due diligence list prior to discharge from the hospital.

Personally, I have learned to become very conservative about transfusions. Unless the patient is going to die without it, I try to be frugal with blood products and teach my students the same. Over time, the medical community has overcome its romance with transfusions and uses them more sparingly, a wise and prudent change. Just like we discovered HIV, it is possible that decades from now we might discover diseases that are unknown today. We might find tiny fragments of proteins in the blood that sneak into the nooks and crevices of cellular tissues to wreak havoc with the immune system, or disrupt barriers not meant to be porous, or produce inflammation that could mess with the physiological framework of the human body and cause fatal disorders. The patient may look pinker than before that transfusion and feel better too, but the nature of medicine is such that learning from the whole Jehovah's Witness experience to harvest an expedient teaching moment for future caregivers should be a crucial goal of clinical educators, lest we disrepute the Hippocratic oath of *primum non nocere*—first do no harm. This holds true not just for transfusions but also for all kinds of medical treatment—drugs, tests, surgeries, diagnostic procedures, and so on. Often, less is more.

On the other hand, in our effort to follow the oath quite literally, we may occasionally cause harm by *withholding* treatment in the mistaken belief that the treatment itself will be detrimental to the patient because of side effects or other reasons. In such cases, we may rationalize with ourselves that not treating or undertreating is better than adequately treating, even though the clinical setting may be appropriate for it. This may originate from the lack of experience of physicians, a fear of "overusing" the power that we have to prescribe drugs, an anxiety about the patient getting an incriminating side effect, or just plain indifference.

What happens to patients when we do that? For example, when we underprescribe pain medications after surgery or injury, or undertreat withdrawal symptoms from alcohol, cocaine, or heroin, how does it disrupt the ecosystem that is meticulously built within the confines of the hospital walls to provide the most appropriate care? Do the patients just randomly check out of the hospital or abscond in search of those drugs and alcohol? Do they hurt themselves in the process? Do they continue to suffer stoically within the hospital until they can go home? How does it harm the hospital, health systems, and providers? Or perhaps it doesn't really matter when we let sick patients suffer by withholding the treatment they deserve to mitigate their suffering—they are powerless anyway. This is a disturbing thought.

Doctors are often accused of prescribing too much medication, some of which definitely causes incredible harm. But no one ever talks about doctors prescribing *too little* medication. It happens more often than we care to admit. Patients sometimes leave against medical advice, because they do not get what they want from doctors. Checking out like this is usually dangerous for the patient. Let's see how.

CHAPTER 5
REALITY CHECK OF CHECKING OUT

M r. Willie Jones disliked going to the county-hospital emergency room. The wait was long, the waiting room was overcrowded, the front desk staff was often rude, and there was no food available except in the hospital cafeteria, which was closed by 6:00 p.m. Over the last decade, he had gone to the emergency room a handful of times, and things were always the same. The doctors were the only reason he still chose this hospital for medical care—they were some of the best clinicians he had met, and he knew he would be well taken care of. As a bonus, they were much nicer than those at the other hospitals near his home.

This time was no different. He had three episodes of rectal bleeding in the last two days, and persuaded by his sister, who lived in another city. He caught the bus that took him to the train station from where he rode the pink line to the medical district. After four hours of twiddling his thumbs, the triage nurse called his name, and he was escorted to one of the examining rooms in the back where he waited another half an hour before the emergency-room doctor knocked on the door. After taking his history and completing the physical examination, the doctor advised him to be admitted to the hospital for further tests to evaluate the source of the bleeding, which could be serious, like colon cancer. Though he was strongly averse to this idea, he grudgingly agreed to it, on the condition that he would be discharged as soon as all the tests were completed.

I met him in the emergency room after he was admitted under my service. The rest of my team of medical students, interns, and residents had already evaluated him by then. He was somewhat annoyed at the same questions being asked by so many people and just wanted to rest.

"I am going to go home tomorrow, right, Doc?" he asked me.

"Only if all the tests are done and the reports are normal, Mr. Jones," I said.

I was skeptical that this would happen. The county system did not work smoothly like a well-oiled machine—more like a creaky engine that had to be cranked up repeatedly. Mr. Jones was sixty-two years old and had mild anemia on his blood tests. The triad of rectal bleeding, anemia, and male gender was an absolute indication for a colonoscopy to examine for colon cancer. If that test were normal, he would need an upper endoscopy to look for diseases in the esophagus, stomach, and proximal small intestine. The latter could be done later as an outpatient procedure, as there was no emergent indication. But a colonoscopy was a must before he could be discharged. At the county hospital, the wait for an outpatient colonoscopy could be up to a year so an inpatient was always preferable.

I admitted him to the medical floor and discussed the plan of action with my team. We would start the prep for a colonoscopy tonight. He would remain on a liquid diet all day and then no food after dinner. He was given four tablets of a laxative and one gallon of Golytely to drink over the next several hours. Golytely is a bowel-cleansing solution that would clear out his colon to allow the colonoscope to visualize the lumen for pathological conditions like cancer, abnormal blood vessels, ulcers, polyps, and so on. Everyone hoped that there would be a spot for him tomorrow in the gastroenterologist's list. The intern was directed to seek out the specialist personally and discuss the options.

The next morning I met Mr. Jones during resident rounds and discussed his overnight stay. He had several episodes of diarrhea after the Golytely but no bleeding. He was very hungry. He wished he could eat a sandwich. We advised him gently not to do so as he was lucky he had a spot later in the afternoon for the colonoscopy.

"I have to stay hungry until three p.m.?" he asked sourly.

"Yes, sir, but I promise I will get you a nice burger afterward," said my very competent resident.

"And then you could possibly go home," I added for good measure.

A couple of hours later the intern paged me. The nurse had found Mr. Jones eating something. Apparently, he had sneaked in a chicken sandwich from his roommate, though he vehemently denied it. The colonoscopy was canceled and postponed for the next day, as he had to be NPO for the procedure—nil per oral. I went down to meet with him and had a long discussion. He was apologetic initially, attributing his action to not having eaten solid food for almost two days. Then he became a little belligerent—he wanted to smoke. Of course, hospital rules did not allow that.

"Doc, I can't eat. I can't smoke. You gotta cut me some slack."

"I will order a nicotine patch for you. It will help control your urges to smoke," I said.

"Nah, those patches don't work. I have used them before. I need a cigarette."

"Well, you cannot smoke in the hospital."

"Then I would like to go home. Please discharge me." He was adamant.

Leaving against medical advice (AMA)—a complex situation that provokes a range of reactions among doctors—is not an infrequent occurrence faced by health-care providers. If the patient has been difficult, there is relief. If he or she is homeless, there is concern. If he or she is very sick, there is anxiety. In the case of Mr. Jones, who was neither difficult, nor homeless, nor horribly sick, I felt that we would squander a valuable opportunity to evaluate him for a serious disease. It was almost impossible to schedule a colonoscopy within twenty-four hours of admitting a patient. He had been lucky twice since we were able to reschedule it a second time for the next day.

"Mr. Jones, please stay for one more day. I promise, you will be able to go home tomorrow. We must ensure you don't have cancer." I found myself cajoling him to stay.

"Doc, I'll stay if I can smoke. You can let me go out of the hospital for ten minutes."

"I don't think I can," I said. Not only was it against hospital policy, I suspected he would walk out and just go home if we let him out of sight, another statistic lost to follow up with no structured access to primary care. He could have early colon cancer that was curable, but if he neglected care, then it could spread and have a worse prognosis.

"OK, give me something to eat then." He shrugged.

"Well, since you have the procedure tomorrow, you have to be on a liquid diet today."

Even as I said these words, I found myself shaking my head in disbelief! Starve the poor guy again for another day? We were setting him up to fail! I felt a twinge of guilt. He was never going to agree to stay another night without food, without a cigarette, more diarrhea, and interrupted sleep.

I had an idea.

"Mr. Jones, give me a few minutes; let me figure something out," I assured him and stepped out of his room. Maybe I could escort him out of the hospital to the curb and let him smoke quickly there. I would not let him out of my sight for a second and then escort him back to his room. I paged the chief resident on call and asked her if it was OK to do so. She was stumped. She had never faced such a scenario. I thanked her and politely hung up. I was going to do it. I was ready to face the consequences of my actions but not willing to give up on him.

Mr. Jones was excited to hear of the plan. He had a pack of cigarettes with him and borrowed a lighter from his roommate. He was in his own clothes and not wearing a hospital gown. We walked to the elevator and went down together. We tried to look casual. No one noticed us. We stepped out of the doors and found a clear area on the curb. I walked away a few steps to give him some privacy. He lit his cigarette and puffed heartily. Then he turned and stopped a stranger walking past us. He offered him a cigarette and they started to chat. I guess smokers like to smoke in company! I never took my eyes off him. I escorted him back to his room when he was done fifteen minutes later. He promised to stay the night and get the procedure done tomorrow. I heaved a sigh of relief and walked back to the nursing station. I was not going to tell anyone except my resident. No harm done, I thought; why complicate matters? All I wanted at that moment was for him to get the colonoscopy safely the next day.

Next morning during resident rounds, we found Mr. Jones still sleeping. He mumbled that he was ready for the procedure later that day. The whole team was walking on eggshells to avoid saying or doing anything that would rock the boat. An hour later, the resident paged me. They could not find Mr. Jones. I hurried to his room. We spoke to the nurse who said he had left, as he "could not take it anymore and just had to eat." He did not sign any requisite AMA papers. My team and I felt disheartened. In county lingo, the patient had absconded. There was not much left for us to do. We do not pursue patients after they abscond from the hospital. All we could do was pray for him.

This is one of many eventful incidents regarding patients absconding from hospitals. Patients leaving against medical advice from emergency rooms is common and a recognized problem. According to Dr. Mathew Delaney, assistant professor of emergency medicine at the University of Alabama at Birmingham, only 0.1 percent of ER patients left AMA in 1992. However, that number has gone up to 2 percent in recent times. In some studies, up to

6 percent of ER patients in the inner city hospitals leave AMA. As the patient safety officer at a safety-net hospital, I was assigned to study the patterns and predictors of patients who abscond from the medical and surgical floors (not ER) after admission, with the strategic goal of implementing initiatives that could reduce absconding, considered a high-risk event deleterious to patient safety. In my research about patients leaving against medical advice, I found that the negative consequences of such events are manifold—poor health outcomes because of fragmented care and confounding diagnoses, increased cost of care because of readmissions and advanced disease, danger to self and others, increased demands on staff time, anxiety in health-care providers, and high medicolegal risks. The terminology used to identify such patients was also confusing—elopement, wandering patient, runaway patient, LAMA, and so on. A fair measure of research has been done on patients leaving against medical advice. Most of the current literature was from psychiatric hospitals. In our institution, we defined absconders as a subset of AMA patients who left hospital premises without signing the requisite paperwork. In literal terms, these patients just got up and walked out of the hospital without staff sanction, a proper discharge, medications, instructions for follow-up, or appointments. There was scant research on this subgroup of patients. My aim was to understand the rationale behind such behavior and perhaps develop a patient profile that would trigger a series of events that could allow a multidisciplinary team to hone in quickly on a potential absconder and prevent absconding.

When I was admitted for major abdominal surgery at a private university hospital in Chicago, I was given a patient-controlled morphine pump on the first day that I used copiously to control my pain. On the second day, this pump was taken away, and I was prescribed oral Norco and ibuprofen. I hadn't even started drinking liquids. My abdomen was distended from gas because of paralytic ileus—a term that describes the inactive bowels after surgery. I had an eight-inch surgical incision and felt like an organ had been viciously ripped out from my body. No amount of begging for stronger pain medicines was heard. On the third day, my surgeon visited me to find me sitting in a chair by the bed curled up in agony. She ordered intravenous Toradol, a non-narcotic that worked really well. Her residents later gave me one more injection and then discontinued it, "since it could damage the kidneys." Such poor pain control after a major operation (especially for a doctor) compelled me to wonder how inadequately health-care providers, including perhaps me, must treat the general population, a fact scientifically proven in literature.

The findings from my project confirmed what we already know. We, as physicians, do not do enough when it comes to certain kinds of care like pain control, adequate management of alcohol- and drug-withdrawal symptoms and discharging patients within a quick time frame. We commonly admit patients for intractable pain from causes other than surgery, such as trauma, cancer, musculoskeletal problems, and so on. Insufficient pain control during a hospital admission was found to be one of the major reasons why patients abscond. Similarly, we do precious little for management of symptoms of withdrawal from alcohol or drugs and urges to smoke. At a public hospital—or at any hospital, honestly—patients with long-standing addictions are commonly admitted for other medical or surgical reasons and often suffer from withdrawal. Most of the absconding patients were active users of alcohol, drugs, and cigarettes, and the majority of them were on inadequate withdrawal protocols. As health-care providers, it should be our duty to prescribe a round-the-clock regimen that alleviates symptoms like anxiety, tremors, high blood pressure, and so on. In the case of smokers, an urge to smoke makes patients restless and agitated, and it is a powerful predictor of absconding. If a proper medication regimen is not prescribed in a timely manner either for pain or withdrawal, patients get very uncomfortable and tend to leave the hospital premises to go get a drink, drugs, or a cigarette to counter the withdrawal. Sometimes they return afterward; mostly they do not.

Why do health-care providers do this? There is no hard data on the rationale behind withholding such treatment but it is possible that in our minds, we become judgmental about "addicts" and simply think that they "deserve to suffer," or that they are malingerers and want to manipulate us into giving them their drug of choice. Or, as in my case after my surgery, that the perceived harms from narcotic pain medications are greater than the benefits, even if given briefly for an obviously painful condition. This is clearly not true, and in my role as a teaching-faculty member, I always emphasize to my students the importance of pain control in a hospital. There is no reason why any patient should suffer from pain or symptoms of substance withdrawal within the controlled confines of a hospital where the abuse potential is decidedly the least. These findings from my study led to relevant changes in institutional policy and the implementation of a substance-use-withdrawal protocol embedded as a careset within the electronic medical record that would automatically pop up at intake for every single admitted patient.

Other reasons why patients abscond include delay in procedures and surgeries, dislike for the medical team (rare), and issues with food, like "starving" them prior to a procedure, as in the case of Mr. Jones. At a public hospital, a curious occurrence is the dip in patient load seen on the first of every month. It has been postulated that patients on social security collect their monthly check on this day and either do not keep their scheduled outpatient appointments or check out of the hospital if admitted.

Another system trigger that results in absconding is a delay in completing the discharge process. Historically, we most often discuss the plan of the day with our patients during morning rounds. If we anticipate discharging them, we let them know that they will be able to go home at a certain time. However, before they can actually do so, there is a series of tasks that need to be completed to close the loop on the hospital admission, including prescriptions for medications, a discharge summary, home health arrangements, and so on—things that may delay the actual time when patients can leave the hospital. Any such delays could interfere with patients' plans, like getting a ride home or picking up medications at a pharmacy before it closes, and spur them to abscond. I found this last behavior particularly peculiar until I had to take my son to the emergency room once for persistent high fever. This was at a state-of-the-art private hospital where we were ushered into a room within a few minutes of reaching there, but had to wait two hours before we met the doctor who spent barely five minutes with us before she discharged him home with instructions. It took another two hours before the discharge summary was completed and we were good to go. In the interim, my family was willing to "abscond" rather than wait interminably for the discharge papers! I had to physically hold on to them to prevent them from escaping and understood much better the impatience that people can feel to flee the hospital premises after they have been deemed as recovered or cured by their health-care providers. Socioeconomic issues unique to the vulnerable population, such as a lack of health-care literacy, language barriers, a lack of transportation, fragmented access to medical care, intense family problems, and so on, only augment and intensify this problem.

A particularly worrisome aspect of absconding is readmissions for the same medical problem. Our study revealed that a quarter of them are readmitted within thirty days and three out of four are for the same problem. A similar number are readmitted within sixty to ninety days, a large majority for the same problem. This not only increases the cost of care and the burden on an already overloaded system but also puts the patients at higher risk of getting sicker and dying. A "wandering patient" is one who repeatedly gets admitted and then leaves against medical advice. "Elopement" implies the same as absconding. "Runaway" is the term used for patients who disappear from psychiatric hospitals. However, the derogatory undertone of these terms, including "absconders," has guided a change in the nomenclature of such patients. They are now increasingly being addressed as "left before treatment completed" or "left without being seen." The police departments in most major cities have high-risk criteria for missing people, and hospitals could collaborate with them to identify high-risk elopement criteria to prevent such events. Ideally, a multidisciplinary team should develop a profile for patients at flight risk for early identification so that steps can be taken to meet their needs while they are admitted in the hospital.

After all, absconding can undeniably be categorized as a critical but preventable medical error. In 1999, the Institute of Medicine carried a report on medical errors that had four core messages: the magnitude of harm from medical errors is huge, most errors are the result of system failures and not human failures, stronger reporting systems are necessary, and patient safety needs to be a top national priority. Clearly, all four elements are central to preventing patients from absconding from hospital floors.

An obvious question that arises from this issue is whether absconding patients are different from those who do not abscond and in what way. My study revealed that those who left before treatment was completed were eight times more likely to have a history of alcohol abuse than those who did not, seven times more likely to be a current smoker, and seven and a half times more likely to have abused drugs. Substance abuse in general is widespread and multifactorial—alcohol, smoking, drugs, even food, the newest drug of abuse. It's not just a medical problem. It has devastating social, economic, and psychological repercussions that can affect individuals and their families in an ongoing manner. Alcoholism continues to be a leading addiction disorder all over the world. Besides, it is the root cause of serious consequences like traffic accidents, domestic violence, sexual assaults, and child abuse. Management of this problem has been somewhat stagnant in recent times, and we are not witnessing much in the form of new treatment, modern preventive and diagnostic tools, or comprehensive, public-health programs that are innovative and effective.

On the other hand, there are some novel therapies for smoking, like electronic cigarettes and medications like Chantix. Marijuana, traditionally considered a recreational drug, is now being used to treat a few chronic, disabling medical disorders that have been unresponsive to other treatments—an exciting new movement that is revolutionary in its concept. However, substance abuse is a vexing problem within all population subgroups, and it is critical that dissemination of accurate information related to these controversial therapies is consistent and trustworthy, backed by vigorous scientific data, and endorsed for the correct clinical diagnoses. The cornucopia of random, ambiguous information on the Internet has become just another extraordinary battle in the life of doctors and other health-care providers. We desperately want to win this battle before it becomes a war. A smart choice would be to trust information originating from a health-care expert only. So keep reading.

CHAPTER 6
BATTLING HIGH SPIRITS

"Hi, it's Dr. Pandey. I was paged."

"Hello, Doctor. Let me get Mr. Leonard's nurse for you."

The ward secretary put me on hold. Beethoven's fifth symphony gently coursed through my phone into my ear. The ebbs and flows of the incredible masterpiece seemed to have an ominous note somehow. I could not quite explain it.

"Dr. Pandey? I am so sorry to bother you. I wanted to let you know that Mr. Leonard spiked a fever of one hundred two Fahrenheit. He is a little confused and had an oxygen level of 88 percent, so I put him on a nasal cannula with two liters of oxygen."

I continued to speak to the nurse for a few more minutes, gave her some orders, and said I would check in to see him within the next half hour.

I lived about ten minutes away from the hospital, and it was an easy drive. As I sat behind the wheel, I could not help but think about the first time I met Mr. Leonard—two days ago, on my first day as an independent attending physician in the United States. He was my first patient, assigned to me through the emergency-room roster. He was a fifty-nine-year-old, Caucasian man admitted with acute alcohol intoxication. The ER physician confided that he was a "frequent flyer"—recurrent ER admissions for alcohol-related problems.

To make matters worse, he had vomited blood, most likely from a tear in the esophagus that could have occurred because of the retching motions that occur when alcohol use irritates the stomach lining. He was incoherent when I met him but seemed to improve over the next thirty-six hours. In one of his lucid intervals, he confessed to drinking a pint of vodka daily for most of the last two decades. His father also drank excessively, and one of his brothers had passed away from alcohol addiction.

My concerns about his rapid deterioration were confirmed, and he was eventually transferred to intensive care with a massive empyema—pus in the linings covering the lung that compromised his respiratory status and necessitated intubation and mechanical ventilation. He remained very sick for two weeks, underwent thoracic surgery, and had a slow postoperative recovery. More than once, I thought we would lose him. He had no visitors, as his surviving family members had disowned him because of alcoholism. He had no friends, and he lived in a motel.

But he survived.

On the day of discharge, we had a long conversation about his drinking habits.

"You almost died, you know. Time to think about quitting."

"Yes, doctor. This is it. Never again."

I believed him. Over the next year, I met him once a month in my office. I found out that he was a hilarious person. He made me and the staff laugh so much that we always looked forward to his visits. He swore he was not drinking. At every visit, I suggested he seek help with alcoholics anonymous or similar support groups. I offered to get him connected with rehabilitation services and social workers who could help him with his addiction. He refused all such services and insisted he could quit all by himself, as he was committed to abstinence and full recovery.

"I would never do that, Doctor, not anymore."

"That's wonderful," I said. We had the same conversation every time.

"Doc, I wanted to ask you about something." Three months later, he had some excitement in his life other than alcohol.

"Sure, Mr. Leonard, anything."

"I found someone. And I need some help."

"What do you mean? Like a lady friend?"

"Yes. Do you think you could prescribe me some of those blue pills?" He was bashful—a whole new demeanor.

"Of course! I am so happy for you!" I was excited, felt thrilled that he had turned his life around to actually be in a relationship. I felt a personal victory—I had reformed a die-hard alcoholic. In my young career, this was incredible.

In another of his visits, he left a message for me with my receptionist when he was checking out. He did not want to tell me himself.

"Tell Dr. Pandey that she is slipping." I was confused. What did he mean?

"I think he meant that your slip is showing under your skirt," my receptionist said laughingly. I looked down and saw what she was talking about. I felt embarrassed, but amused at the same time. Mr. Leonard was incorrigible!

To me, interactions like these indicated that he was slowly but surely regaining his normal composure and moving toward normal life independent of alcohol. He never missed an appointment. He bought little gifts for us. He never had to go to the ER for any reason. He was diligently following all my instructions including visits to specialists and tests if needed. He called back when we left him a voice mail to discuss something. But he always refused any rehabilitative support. In my mind, he was a recovered alcoholic.

A year or so later, paramedics brought him to the ER in an incoherent state. His blood alcohol level was very high. A subsequent upper endoscopy revealed acute inflammation of the lining of his esophagus and stomach, caused by chronic alcohol use. He had not told me the truth—he was indeed back to his old drinking habits. He had to have been drinking for a while. This was not the result of a single binge episode. I suspect he never wanted to quit at all.

As a newly minted doctor, I felt incredibly disappointed. Why did he do this? What made him go back to drinking? How can he put himself at risk of serious illness after his experiences? It was baffling to me at that time. I was aware that there was a high risk of relapse because of his family history. Many questions came to my mind. How is alcoholism inherited from generation to generation? Is it genetically determined? Why don't we see all siblings suffer equally? How can we know which offspring will become an addict if a parent is an alcoholic?

In wine there is wisdom, in beer there is freedom,
in water there is bacteria.

—Benjamin Franklin

Any doctor will tell you that alcohol-related hospital visits are common, and physicians get to see such patients frequently irrespective of their chosen specialty. Intoxication, withdrawal, seizures, cirrhosis of liver, bleeding, encephalopathy, and jaundice are some of the alcohol-related problems that need emergent care. Death because of alcohol-related diseases is common. The fifth edition of the *Diagnostic and Statistical Manual of Mental Disorders* (*DSM-5*), issued by the American Psychiatric Association in 2013, termed alcoholism as "alcohol use disorder" (AUD) and combines the prior classification into alcohol abuse and alcohol dependence. Eleven criteria have been listed, and the presence of two or more receives a diagnosis of AUD. Craving to use alcohol was added as a new criterion, and legal problems because of alcohol use, a criterion in *DSM-4*, was eliminated.

For decades, we have known that family history plays an important role in alcoholism. However, a genetic basis has been questioned in the past, and exposure to parental alcohol-related behaviors has been deemed as a predictor of children veering toward alcohol abuse. Those with a positive family history of chronic alcohol abuse tend to have a higher risk of similar drinking habits irrespective of adverse life experiences. In fact, children of alcoholics are four times more likely to have alcohol-related problems. However, the National Institute on Alcohol Abuse and Alcoholism clearly states that half the risk for alcoholism originates in genes. The other half is determined by environmental factors and the interplay between genetic and environmental factors. Furthermore, the success of alcoholism treatment may also depend on genetics, at least partly. Presence of a specific gene may determine whether a patient will respond to a certain treatment. Deeper understanding of these genetic factors may be critical in prescribing the most appropriate treatment that will result in the best clinical outcome.

All of us know that we tend to gravitate toward people who have something in common with us. Shared interests are a way of breaking the ice and forging relationships. Mostly, this is expected to have a positive outcome, because conventional wisdom dictates that such partnerships are more likely to be successful. However, it can be a destructive liaison. It has been scientifically proven repeatedly that people who have common *behaviors*, especially substance abuse, are attracted to each other and tend to marry each other more frequently. "Assortative mating" is an anthropological trait that is defined as discrete nonrandom reproductive pairing of people who have common physical, psychological, or other traits that are genetically linked. Children of such couples are likely to inherit these common genetic traits at a higher rate than otherwise. Thus if two people with similar alcohol-related lifestyles mate or marry, their children are at considerably higher risk of alcoholism genetically as well as environmentally, being exposed to two parents with alcoholism. This is likely to affect successive generations too and thus whole population. The tendency for mate selection based on similar traits helps in understanding the genetic contribution to alcoholism and is very helpful in predicting the clinical prognosis too. Person A, who has both parents with AUD has a worse prognosis than person B with one parent with AUD, not just because the child watches both of his parents drink but also because he or she inherited the trait from both. Family history has also been described as a predictor of those who are more likely to relapse after a liver transplant for alcoholic cirrhosis of the liver. The risk increases if both parents are alcoholics, another pitfall of assortative mating. I don't have any information on whether Mr. Leonard's mother had a history of AUD. But he may have been doomed from the outset if she did.

The occurrence of adverse events early in life enhances the risk of alcoholism later in life, though it is not inevitable. However, neither a family history nor a troubled household with alcoholic parent(s) can guarantee that the children will suffer from alcohol use disorder. The risk is certainly higher, but it is impossible to predict 100 percent which offspring will be afflicted with AUD. Many children from such families do not abuse alcohol. This is where science gets somewhat unclear. I have witnessed many such patients who have a family history but do not drink excessively themselves. In a study done on twins (identical and fraternal) it was found that the decision to seek treatment for alcoholism was substantially determined by genetic factors too. Alcohol abusers may understand that they have a problem and seek or not seek help based on their genetic makeup. This finding helps explain why we see so many patients with alcoholism who seek health care only emergently for alcohol-related complications like intoxication, withdrawal, bleeding, or neurological symptoms, instead of proactively seeking help for rehabilitation. In short, at least some alcoholics do not want to quit at all, no matter how seriously their health may be affected. Mr. Leonard probably falls into this subset.

Culturally, Americans suffer more from AUD than citizens of several other countries, possibly because in the United States, alcohol has been historically consumed mostly for the purpose of intoxication. Among Muslims and Jews, drunkenness is frowned upon, even considered a sin, and moderate consumption of alcohol with meals is an accepted practice in some of these cultures.

Ulysses Grant, the eighteenth president of the United States and the face on the fifty-dollar bill, was a well-known drunk. He got fired from his position in the army for drinking excessively. However, during the Civil War, he enlisted in the army again and directed it to victory under Abraham Lincoln's leadership while continuing his major dalliance with whiskey. Lincoln was aware of his addiction, but in a vigorous show of support, he once inquired about the brand of whiskey Grant drank, so that he could send a vat to his other army generals! Winston Churchill's passion for alcohol is legendary. We do not know whether he earned his reputation as a die-hard alcoholic or he actively encouraged the rumor. He is once known to have said that he drank before, during, and after meals, and he supposedly began his day with a drink for decades. President Roosevelt is known to have enjoyed an alcoholic camaraderie with him during his visits to the White House in what has been notoriously termed "Winston Hours," a session of unlimited inebriation that required the president to recover over the next three days with a total of thirty hours of nightly sleep!

Ernest Hemingway was another American who was addicted to alcohol. He apparently wrote much of his excellent literary work in a drunken haze. The Dutch artist Vincent van Gogh blamed alcohol for his "madness" though he had an underlying serious psychiatric disorder. Both of these incredibly creative artists committed suicide by shooting themselves.

Recent studies have revealed that a positive family history may be a predictor of negative personality traits like antisocial behavior, poor impulse control, negative moods, and so on, and it has been linked to clinical depression. Alcoholics Anonymous (AA), which has more than two million active members, was cofounded by Bill Wilson, an alcoholic who described alcohol as the elixir of life. Other famous people who died because of alcohol-related illness include Alexander the Great, Boris Yeltsin, and Joseph McCarthy.

For those who want to be proactive and protect themselves because of their family history, simple suggestions and a common-sense approach work the best. Complete abstinence from alcohol would be ideal but perhaps not feasible. A three-pronged tactic should include avoidance of early-age drinking, moderate drinking habits as an adult, and transparency with your health-care provider from the get-go. The National Association for Children of Alcoholics is a safe place to seek help. There is a toll-free telephone line to call and choose resources available (1-888-55-4COAS).

An ideal future for children of alcoholic parents would be somewhat similar to cancer genetics:

- Availability of tests to determine gene mutations or other specific inherited genes
- Validated, computerized calculation tools to estimate the genetic risk of alcoholism
- Evidence-based recommendations for screening for primary care physicians
- Prevention strategies for patients meant to be employed as early as adolescence and young adulthood

A simple online model called the Gail Model that assesses a five-year and lifetime risk for breast cancer based on personal and family history can calculate the risk for someone who has a strong family history of cancer. It takes barely a few minutes to complete and provides a guideline for providers to recommend an overarching prevention plan, including MRI of the breasts and/or chemotherapy with drugs like tamoxifen. A similar instrument for alcoholism may be an excellent way to precisely calculate risk in people with a family history of alcoholism that would reinforce the physician's assessment for the patient. It sounds considerably better to say, "You have an X percent risk and need Y treatment," than to say, "Hey, you need to *not* drink at all because your parents drank all your beer!" Patients follow heed when you give them numbers to put it all in context, rather than ambiguous advice. Imagine if I could have calculated Mr. Leonard's risk scientifically to say, "Since you have an X percent risk, you will benefit enormously from going to rehab, or attending AA meetings, or taking a certain test every week." It just sounds a lot more credible and convincing.

Unfortunately, Mr. Leonard continued to drink and was admitted intermittently for emergent care. He expressed guilt at his addiction and at "letting me down." I eventually lost track of him, and I suspect he may have passed away from alcohol-related complications. He once gave me a tiny glass cherub with wings and told me that I was his guardian angel. I still have it safely ensconced in my living room where it remains a wistful reminder that perhaps I was the one who failed him. Could I have done more? It's a question that all doctors ask themselves regularly—what more can we do for our patients? This constant quest to improve medical care has led to considerable innovation in medicine, some groundbreaking and radical, others not so much. Some work well but may have their own risks. And occasionally, we may replace one harmful habit or drug with another one that ostensibly seems harmless but may not be so. For example, smoking and electronic cigarettes—do we have a beauty or a beast?

CHAPTER 7

VAPING, NOT SMOKING

Dee Harris was a fifty-six-year-old woman with multiple medical problems, one of which was heavy smoking—she had smoked one to two packs per day for forty years. She had early signs of emphysema with shortness of breath on walking more than four or five blocks, occasional wheezing, especially in the cold, and a mild dry cough that was most prominent in the morning. She used an albuterol inhaler as needed. She had numerous chest X-rays and lung function tests that indicated that the damage from the smoke had begun to affect her lungs, though it was still in the very early stages.

Dee understood very well that cigarette smoke was her number one enemy, and if she did not quit, she was likely going to get a progressive disease and might end up requiring oxygen at home. On the other hand, if she stopped smoking now, there was still a chance for her to improve her lung health over the next decade or so.

I met with Dee every two to three months in my office for monitoring her medical problems. She was a model patient in many ways. She never missed an appointment with me and always followed directions for blood tests, X-rays, and other investigations that her specialists or I requested. She was intelligent and always pleasant. I looked forward to seeing her in my clinic. In the tough world of a safety-net county hospital with an excessively high burden of disease, I considered her an "easy" patient for the reasons above. As a cherry on the icing, she had a wry sense of humor that was self-deprecating with a "whatcha-gonna-do" drollness that made me laugh. I knew she would have all her medicines with her for reconciliation. I knew she would have completed every test that I requested in the last visit. I knew that most of her medical conditions would be well under control.

Except for one—smoking cigarettes. In spite of several efforts to quit, she had been unable to stop smoking and at times just didn't want to. She was unemployed, had no health insurance, and lived on a disability check in other people's homes—initially with her long-term boyfriend, and later in the basement of her brother's house. Smoking was the one guilty pleasure of her life. She didn't want to give it up even though she understood the repercussions very well.

Following the smoking cessation guidelines, I spent time talking to her about quitting in every single visit. We went over her options—nicotine-replacement therapy with the nicotine patch, gum, and spray; Chantix, the new medication that was very popular and moderately effective; and Wellbutrin, the conventional antidepressant used for smoking cessation. I discussed behavior modification strategies in detail—delay smoking right after waking up; substitute with other things like celery, carrots, straw, toothpick, and so on for cigarettes; keep herself busy when she has the urge to smoke; throw away the ashtrays and cigarette packs in her home; stop smoking inside the house, and so on. At different times, she tried every one of those suggestions except Chantix—it was too expensive and the county-hospital pharmacy did not have it on their formulary.

She still continued to smoke at least one pack of cigarettes a day.

Until one day, she arrived in my clinic for her regular appointment, and before I could say much, she whipped out what looked like a slimly built pen, put it in her mouth, and drew on it, exhaling smoke through her mouth. I was horrified! I had a patient in my office smoking right in front of me, in the room assigned specifically for smoking-cessation counseling! Not only was it personally appalling to me, I was also afraid that if my supervisor witnessed this in the clinic, it would lead to plenty of hand-wringing and admonishment. Afterward, I learned that it was vapor and not smoke that Dee had exhaled.

This was my first experience with electronic cigarettes, or e-cigarettes. Later, Dee told me how she had ordered it online after a friend recommended it to her. She had been trying to replace her regular cigarettes with it and thought she was succeeding in cutting back. She felt very enthusiastic about it. She sent me an e-mail with a link to a site that I could pass on to my other patients. She even gave me a discount code for them.

This was several years ago when electronic cigarettes had just been introduced into the market. Since then they have become quite popular among smokers, raking in billions of dollars in global sales. It remains somewhat of a mystery to many people, with skeptics decrying it as a scam and not without harm. Supporters, on the other hand, assert that they have been able to stop or reduce smoking using an EC when all other options had failed. Like it or not, its popularity cannot be ignored. The *Oxford Dictionary*, which claims to keep up with the times in linguistics, added the word "vape" in 2014—"to inhale and exhale the vapor produced by an electronic cigarette."

Burden of Disease

Cigarette smoking remains the number one preventable cause of disease in the world with six-million deaths annually caused by tobacco use. More than four-hundred-thousand deaths a year in the United States are attributed to it directly or indirectly, costing approximately $300 billion every year. Most morbidity and deaths are from cancer and cardiovascular disease. Smoking causes almost 90 percent of lung cancer globally, and it is the most common cause of cancer deaths in both men and women in the United States. Secondhand smoke has also been shown to be deleterious and a cause of lung cancer. Thirdhand smoke, a relatively recently recognized phenomenon, is the residue left behind after the cigarette smoke has disappeared. It lingers on the walls, furniture, carpet, clothing, nails, and hair, and it combines with other indoor pollutants to form harmful chemicals that are equally injurious. They persist for months or years and are difficult to measure or eradicate. They can cause cancer too, but the real concern that the health-care providers and researchers are anxious is that it may affect our genetic makeup and cause generational harm that could begin with babies and children being the early victims.

Contrary to popular understanding, smoking has been implicated in twelve types of cancer including lung, pancreatic, esophageal, gastric, urinary bladder, kidney, mouth, larynx, liver, cervix, colon, and rectum, as well as acute myeloid leukemia (https://www.cancer.gov/about-cancer/causes-prevention/risk/tobacco/cessation-fact-sheet). These cancers together cause almost half the deaths in the United States. In fact, it affects almost every organ in the body, one way or another. Smoking also causes emphysema; chronic bronchitis; ulcers in the gastrointestinal system; stroke; heart attack; osteoporosis; erectile dysfunction; pregnancy-related illnesses like infertility, preterm birth, low birth weight, miscarriages, and so on; and general thickening of the arteries called atherosclerosis because of repeated cellular damage from smoke. Buerger's disease is a unique condition caused almost exclusively by smoking that affects the blood supply to the arteries of the legs and sometimes arms. It mostly affects young male smokers between twenty to forty years old but can be seen in women and older people too. Smokeless tobacco is also associated with it. The patient suffers from intractable pain, and in severe cases can get ulcers and gangrene of the toes and fingers that may need amputation. The only known treatment for this condition is smoking cessation.

The overall loss of quality of life is enormous, and the contribution of smoking to disability worldwide cannot be overemphasized. Such a high and widespread burden of disease linked to smoking needs to be addressed constantly by health-care providers and researches in a sustained effort to somehow find ways to help smokers quit (primary prevention) as well as diagnose and treat diseases caused by it (secondary prevention). The powerful tobacco industry that spends almost $10 billion on advertising and marketing tobacco every year, has failed to engage with the medical community, public-health experts, or the government in legitimate health-related concerns in a collaborative manner. According to the Centers for Disease Control, in 2011, 70 percent smokers wanted to quit and more than 40 percent had attempted to quit in the past year. Electronic cigarettes have thus found support in an eager, and sometimes desperate, clientele of patients and occasionally providers, who are willing to try any remedy that can lessen their dependence on cigarettes.

What Are Electronic Cigarettes?

Electronic nicotine delivery systems (ENDS) are an assortment of devices that are used to dispense nicotine to smokers in forms other than regular cigarettes. One of these devices is the electronic cigarette, a slimly built tool that resembles a regular cigarette in its looks and use. It is battery-operated and contains nicotine, which is the main ingredient of addiction in cigarettes. This nicotine mixes with flavors and chemicals, such as propylene glycol, formaldehyde, and acetaldehyde, and is contained in a liquid form within a cartridge. The concoction is delivered to the user through a heating device called the vaporizer in a vapor form instead of smoke. On inhaling, the vaporizer is activated to deliver an aerosol of nicotine, unlike in a regular cigarette where nicotine is inhaled by burning tobacco leaves. There are currently more than 450 varieties of electronic cigarettes in the market to choose from; some of them shaped like a pen, flash drive, or other commonly used items. Almost half of all smokers in the United States have tried electronic cigarettes and 4 percent use them on a regular basis. There is neither robust data on whether electronic cigarettes are safe, effective, and appropriate as a smoking-cessation device, nor has a cost-benefit analysis been done.

Pros

This exotic tool is being extolled as the best thing to have happened to smokers who want to quit. The rationale is that smoke is considered decidedly more injurious to health than vapor since it contains harmful toxins like tar that cause tissue damage, including carcinogens that cause cancer. The pleasurable effects of smoking are attributed to nicotine, which is not considered a carcinogenic chemical, and using it in electronic cigarettes is deemed to be safer. An electronic cigarette satisfies many habits other than the nicotine craving—holding the cigarette in the hand, the sensation of a cigarette between the lips, the habit of swinging the cigarette to the mouth, the inhaling and exhaling of smoke, and so on. They can be used in smoke-free zones like schools and colleges unlike regular cigarettes, a substantial value to smokers.

Cons
Electronic cigarettes have not been conclusively shown to be of benefit in smoking cessation in existing small studies and have low efficacy, if any at all, in helping smokers quit completely for any length of time. The manifold concerns expressed against them include the idea that electronic cigarettes may merely be a fad that makes smoking socially acceptable. It may also attract nonsmokers to start smoking in the belief that it is harmless. But mostly the worry stems from the possibility that electronic cigarettes may weaken the motivation of a serious smoker to completely quit. The debate explores the possibility that while the mode of delivery may change, smokers continue their addiction to nicotine. The inclination to undermine the harms of electronic cigarettes is an alarming trend by experts in smoking cessation, likening it to a mere Band-Aid on a serious underlying addiction to nicotine. Additional harms include nicotine toxicity and the damaging effects of the other components like formaldehyde and acetaldehyde, which could be cancer producing too. Long-term adverse effects are largely unknown. The cartridges in electronic cigarettes that contain the nicotine-laden liquid are refillable and may be used for other drugs.

Another major concern has been that using electronic cigarettes may reduce cigarette smoking but not discontinue it entirely, resulting in concurrent use of both, a practice that could be a predictor of a longer duration of cigarette smoking. A person who uses both may continue to smoke longer over time, erroneously believing that reducing the number of cigarettes smoked daily mitigates the risk for disease. However, it is more harmful overall to have smoked *longer in time* than the *number* of cigarettes a day, thus clearly enhancing bad outcomes with more disease and death. It is too early to quantify such risks and ongoing research is awaited. Simultaneous use increases the risk of nicotine toxicity as well.

Regulatory Control
Any product that affects our health should ideally be under some sort of regulatory control through policies and procedures. Currently, the Food and Drug Administration does not consider EC under its purview of legislation. Promoters of electronic cigarettes disagree with introducing quality control regulations since it does not contain any ingredients of tobacco and is not sold as a tobacco product like regular cigarettes. In spite of all the attention as a smoking-cessation device, it is not recognized for any medically approved therapeutic use in the United States, though Britain very recently recognized it as a relevant tool for smoking cessation. A few small studies comparing electronic cigarettes to regular cigarettes have not reported any serious side effects from them, but most of these studies were done over three to six months only and long-term data are not available.

There is a clear concern for minors using electronic cigarettes. In the absence of any age-related statute by a governing body, they can obtain electronic cigarettes from various sources, including stores and online sales. The fruity flavors mixed with nicotine, as well as its ambiguous reputation, attract teenagers and young adults. As noted earlier, they can be used without restrictions in smoke-free zones like schools and colleges. This kind of behavior carries many risks, two of which are the most worrisome: (1) users of electronic cigarettes may "upgrade" to using regular cigarettes and (2) nicotine may have a detrimental impact on the still growing brains of adolescents. In pregnant women, nicotine can affect the fetal-brain growth too, and pregnant women should not use any form of nicotine. Other chemicals in the liquid may be potentially harmful to the fetus. There are no statutory warnings on electronic cigarettes similar to cigarettes that may caution these vulnerable populations against using them.

These concerns violate the core messages about tobacco control such as "don't start" and "quit if you do." Furthermore, the ENDS market is gradually being taken over by the tobacco industry, which has been eager to get a piece of the pie. This heralds a sinister trend that could seriously undermine any public-health effort to convey accurately the harms from EC.

As far as Dee was concerned, the electronic cigarettes helped her reduce her daily use of cigarettes by a few. She was never able to transition completely because she fell gravely ill and had to be admitted to the hospital. She was diagnosed with a severe pneumonia, which was certainly a result of the damage done to her lungs from smoking. She remained in intensive care for a day, and X-rays and CT scans revealed a lung mass. When I saw the scans, I was sure that she had lung cancer, again a consequence of long-standing smoking. The pulmonary specialists agreed with me. A bronchoscopy was performed that was not very helpful, as the mass was too deep to be biopsied. The cardiothoracic surgeons had to perform an open biopsy—an incision in the chest wall to access the mass and remove a tiny piece for histopathological examination.

While the biopsy results were pending, Dee suffered a complication from the procedure on the telemetry floor—a pneumothorax, a collection of air in between the linings of the lung that caused it to collapse. She went into acute respiratory failure and had to be transferred back to intensive care where a chest tube was inserted to remove the air and reexpand her lung. Throughout this ordeal, Dee remained composed, never losing her sense of humor. Because of her strong smoking history, she was prescribed nicotine patches daily, a treatment that she had used several times in the past without success. Regardless, she never had any urges to smoke during her entire hospital admission, an interesting phenomenon commonly seen even in excessive smokers. It is believed that the clean hospital ambience and absence of the odor of cigarettes are at least partially responsible for this. A few days later, the final biopsy report was a welcome surprise—no cancer, just scar tissue, probably from a prior infection. Dee was discharged to a skilled-nursing facility after three weeks and went home after another three weeks there. The pain and suffering were a nightmare that she endured stoically. The upside? She never smoked another cigarette. Sometimes you have to almost die to still be alive.

CHAPTER 8
HASHING THE HASHISH MYTH

The six-month-old baby in the arms of her father continued to have jerking movements of the whole body for several minutes as I watched the screen of my television in growing horror. There was no way to stop these intractable seizures when they occurred. Dravet syndrome, a congenital form of childhood epilepsy, was the diagnosis given to Charlotte Figi, now a well-known child first seen on Dr. Sanjay Gupta's CNN documentary *Weed*. In spite of being prescribed seven different anticonvulsant medications, she had uncontrolled seizures that had affected her physical and mental growth and caused severe psychosocial and economic harm to her family. In Colorado, a few drops of an oral medicinal solution resolved 99 percent of her seizures per her mother—from three hundred a week to two to three a month. Charlotte walked, talked, ate, and slept in peace—nothing short of a miracle for her and her family. The Stanley Brothers in Colorado, who run C. W. Botanicals that provided this medicine, named the product Charlotte's Web.

The product was a form of marijuana, the most commonly used recreational drug, also known as pot, weed, or grass. Cannabis is the name of the plant and is a term that is used interchangeably with marijuana. It is also one of the most common illegally sold drugs on the street. Tony Dokoupil, a pot dealer in the 1970s, earned millions by smuggling marijuana from the Caribbean and Colombia across the entire East Coast of the United States during what was later termed the golden age of marijuana. Considered as a very smart, risk-taking businessman, he lived in the era of a governmental war on drugs that Richard Nixon enforced. Dokoupil called himself the "Pirate King." He looked down on smugglers of hard drugs like cocaine, though he later became addicted to it himself. Later on in the 1980s, Reagan pushed hard on the war on drugs, especially pot, and such "merchants of marijuana" were treated like terrorists and state enemies. Tony's son went on to write a book called *The Last Pirate* that describes in elaborate detail his father's role in those two decades in establishing marijuana as a lifestyle choice in America, even hailed by many as a laudable effort to "build a better world." The war on drugs continues today, with marijuana possession being a common cause for drug-related arrests.

As I watched the excellent CNN documentary, I found myself wondering if we had been wrong all along about marijuana. After watching *Weed 2* and *Weed 3*, I am convinced that we, the medical community, have done a great disservice to humanity by our failure to correctly estimate the medicinal properties of cannabis, the plant from which marijuana is produced. My recent interview with Joel Stanley, the CEO of C. W. Botanicals, further reinforced this outlook based on the dramatic resurgence of marijuana for medical disorders that was spearheaded by him and his four brothers. The four key concepts about marijuana that I would like to highlight are as follows:

- Addiction to this plant derivative is low.
- No one has ever reported a death because of an overdose from marijuana.

- It has a definite role in symptom relief in several chronic medical disorders.
- Decriminalization (not legalization) of marijuana is a vital issue that leaders, politicians, the judiciary, and advocates need to address.

In 2013, the US Department of Health and Human Services estimated that there were almost six million regular users of marijuana nationwide above the age of twelve who account for 80 percent of marijuana used. Historically, pot usage has been documented as early as 2700 BC in China, from where it spread to the rest of the world. The Chinese were ahead of the world even then. In the nineteenth century, it was used for nausea, labor pains, and joint pains. How wise were health-care providers in olden times! In India, priests and *yogis* of questionable repute have long used it recreationally in different forms like *hashish, charas, ganja,* and *bhang.* In the Hindu festival of colors called *Holi,* celebrated in the spring every year, it is customary to eat or drink *bhang* in any form. It has often been referred to as the "food of the gods." Certain sects of Christianity and Zionism routinely use marijuana in their religious rituals as well as in their personal lives. However, in the early-twentieth century, it started gaining notoriety as a drug of abuse with high addiction potential. It was labeled as a Schedule 1 drug along with LSD and heroin in the Controlled Substances Act of 1970—a drug of high addiction with no known medicinal value. Regardless, its illegal use continued for decades and even garnered a rebellious tag by the hippies of the mid-twentieth century. In the '80s and early '90s, the US government had a Compassionate Use Program for a very limited list of disorders, and patients were enrolled to receive marijuana cigarettes prepared by the government. This program was closed in 1992 for unclear reasons.

Marijuana is most commonly smoked to provide a euphoric feeling and can be eaten in baked goods like brownies or administered in a tablet or liquid form with the same effect. In the Netherlands, there are coffee shops that are legally allowed to serve these baked foods containing low-potency marijuana. Mostly, however, it is illegal all over the world, including in parts of United States. There are three terminologies associated with it that cause confusion: medical marijuana, decriminalization, and legalization.

- "Medical marijuana" is the use of the drug for defined medical disorders under the supervision of a physician and with a prescription. Users have to get a marijuana card, and physicians have to be certified in prescribing it. So far, twenty states have mandated marijuana for medical use in the United States as legal.
- "Decriminalization" is the downgrading of punishment for possession, use, or trade of marijuana, each of which is currently considered a crime with a potential jail sentence of at least one year. With decriminalization, it may just become an infraction with a fine or community service.
- "Legalization" means that possession of a small amount of marijuana by adults for personal use (recreational or medical without a prescription) is deemed legal under state laws. Several states have legalized recreational pot use, including Colorado, Washington, Alaska, Oregon, and most recently, after the presidential elections, California. By the time this book is published, it is highly likely that many other states will also have followed suit to decriminalize or legalize marijuana.

In the last two decades, however, attention has shifted to the medicinal properties of marijuana. As Dr. Sanjay Gupta wrote in an article, the very premise of labeling it as a Schedule 1 drug is shaky. It is based on *insufficient* evidence about its pharmacological properties rather than hardcore evidence about its potential addictive characteristics or dangerous side effects—unlike heroin or LSD, which are clearly harmful in any form. The medical community generally agrees that addiction to marijuana is low (less than 10 percent) and even for those addicted, it is not life threatening as opposed to alcohol, cocaine, or heroin. Cocaine abuse can cause heart attacks, and alcohol intoxication is a common cause of hospitalization. Withdrawal symptoms from alcohol abuse can kill people, but there are no reports of such deaths from marijuana withdrawal. Annually, more than twenty-two hundred people die from alcohol poisoning. According to the Centers for Disease Control, no one has reported a death from a marijuana "overdose."

However, it is not completely harmless, and smoking it can cause the same harms as cigarette smoke. Users may indulge in dangerous activities while high, resulting in injuries or accidents. A curious effect of long term cannabis use has been described in literature as the Cannabis Hyperemesis Syndrome (CHS) in which the user has intractable vomiting after use that is strangely relieved with hot showers. These people tend to spend hours in the bathroom under the shower. A patient with CHS was once admitted under my service. He was almost never found in his bed. The nursing documentation clearly showed that he would take a shower repeatedly and for long periods of time. But compared to other drugs in the same group, as well as alcohol and cigarettes, cannabis is relatively much less harmful. My argument in this context always starts with the fact that it is a plant. This naturally growing ingredient has been around for centuries without any definite documentation anywhere that it is fatal or highly injurious.

In this chapter, I choose not to discuss the issues surrounding the legalization of pot and the concern for abuse, as the legislative and political debate has polarized people. Instead, I want to outline the medical conditions for which marijuana may be useful or has been shown to have positive results in symptom control and/ or disease modification. Traditional medications have proven ineffective for several debilitating conditions. Would it be completely wrong or unethical to try marijuana in such disorders to improve patients' quality of life? There are proponents and opponents. Some quote science to endorse it while others find it challenging to accept or promote a drug traditionally used recreationally, especially one that is widely available illegally. In almost all the disorders named below, further studies are needed to indisputably show specific benefits and less harm. My observations are based on current literature that is inadequate and scientifically weak at best. Anecdotally, cases have been reported that describe medicinal benefits in a compelling way that can treat the symptoms of serious diseases. This description is not intended for the purpose of medical advice for any condition and must not be considered as such. The side effects of using marijuana are many and can be serious. The description below should not be considered as the author's patronage for recreational-drug use in any form.

Seizure Disorder

Charlotte Figi's story inspired many parents across the country to seek marijuana for their children with Dravet disease or similar intractable seizure syndromes. Its effectiveness in controlling seizures in these patients is impressive as described and seen in the *Weed* documentaries. Small clinical trials have shown conflicting reports. One in five patients with epilepsy who smoked marijuana reported a reduction in seizures. Others have reported an increase in frequency or no change. In studies done in the past few decades, there is no objective evidence that it is effective in epilepsy. But individual case reports are hard to ignore. In my opinion, if it relieves intractable seizures even in a few patients, then it is worth to explore this aspect of marijuana. Of course, large clinical trials, which will be convincing are needed to prove effectiveness as a drug of choice. Side effects, especially somnolence in children, can be worrisome, and strict medical supervision is vital. The problem with aggressive research is related to strict mind-boggling regulations that have to do with its status as a controlled substance.

Multiple Sclerosis (MS)

There is definite objective evidence that marijuana reduces spasticity in multiple sclerosis as well as spasm-related pain due to its anti-inflammatory properties. Urinary bladder symptoms, depression, constipation, fecal incontinence, and defecation urgency have also been relieved. Some patients have reported an improvement in sleep. The National MS Society supports patients who are interested in exploring this option to relieve their symptoms and improve their quality of life. Marijuana does not reduce tremors or pain caused by neuropathy in MS, nor does it modify the progression of the underlying disease process. Those MS patients who regularly smoke pot may be at a higher risk for cognitive impairment.

It has been used in various forms for MS like smoking, oral spray, capsules, and so on. Smoking it is harmful for lungs, so the other options are generally preferred. So far, the only form of marijuana that is available by prescription for MS is an oral spray, **Sativex,** manufactured by GW Pharma in the United Kingdom, which has a farm for its production in a hidden location. It is used in MS for spasticity and sleep. Globally, Sativex is available in eleven countries, including the UK, and another thirteen have approved its launch soon, including the United States. Some countries have deemed Sativex too expensive for regular use. Another tablet, called Namisol, is also going to become available soon for use in MS and other conditions below.

Chronic Pain Syndromes

This is the most common use of medical marijuana. Research has consistently shown that if used correctly, it can be valuable for chronic pain syndromes with negligible side effects or risk for addiction. The stigma attached to this indication is immense. Most such users are frivolously branded as "potheads." They are dismissed as using pain as an excuse to get a "high." While there may be a shred of truth in this, marijuana can be of tremendous benefit in many cases like labor pain, intractable headaches or migraines, joint pain from arthritis, cancer pain of different types, pain from spasticity, endometriosis, fibromyalgia, and so on. After robust research of existing literature, the Institute of Medicine (IOM), a highly esteemed peer institution in health care, has deemed that marijuana in any form can cause mild to moderate pain relief on par with codeine. The IOM team considered that patients with anxiety-inducing conditions like AIDS and cancer could possibly benefit the most from marijuana. Others like surgical patients, those with spinal cord injury-related pain and nerve pain, and patients with insomnia could also have good outcomes in terms of pain relief. Older people with pain because of arthritis and other chronic inflammatory conditions are increasingly turning to marijuana with significant relief.

Opiates like morphine and Vicodin that are traditionally prescribed for pain have several problems—significant side effects like nausea and vomiting, sedation, eventual tolerance to pain control properties, potential for serious abuse, and so on. Prescription-painkiller abuse is rampant and kills more people than guns, motor vehicle accidents, or suicide. In those geographical areas where marijuana is available in dispensaries legally, fewer people die from prescription-drug overdose. Marijuana relieves nausea and vomiting, and IOM has recommended clinical trials to conclusively prove if using marijuana with lower doses of opiates for painful conditions could be an effective combination. The IOM was very firm in a statement that any use of marijuana for pain control is best done under fully controlled and supervised conditions.

Amyotrophic Lateral Sclerosis (ALS)

ALS is a degenerative disease of the nerve cells that supply voluntary muscles and is ultimately fatal when muscles of respiration and the diaphragm become too weak to function. Patients initially have muscle spasms, pain, loss of appetite, depression, and they die within three to five years. There is no treatment available currently. Stephen Hawking is one of the most high-profile celebrities who is suffering from this disorder, also known as Lou Gehrig's disease, named after the famous baseball player who was one of the first patients to get this diagnosis. In several case reports, cannabis has been described to relieve pain and muscle spasm, improve breathing by relaxing bronchial muscles, reduce drooling by inhibiting saliva, stimulate appetite, and help in sleep. Its best effect is on depression, which may be relieved for two to three hours. It does not help in speech, swallowing, and sexual dysfunction. Though no clinical trials have been done, there are neurologists and researchers who strongly believe that cannabis might slow down the progression of ALS in humans, based on similar findings in mutant mice that were created with ALS. Among other side effects, one of the dangers of smoking marijuana in ALS is that it may aggravate the already compromised respiratory system and cause death by respiratory failure.

Cathy Jordan, a resident of Florida, was diagnosed with ALS in 1986 and given five years to live. However, she shocked many, as she is still alive after almost three decades and credits marijuana, which she smokes daily, for her health. Her husband grows cannabis at home and makes "joints" for her to smoke, since it is legal to do so in Florida now. Interestingly, most of her doctors are either retired or dead, and the man who provided her with her first marijuana cigarette was arrested and sent to life imprisonment for growing cannabis illegally! Such anecdotal evidence has been reported frequently. Currently, medical marijuana is legally available for use in ALS in six states in the United States: Arizona, Florida, Maine, Michigan, New Jersey, and New Mexico. The ALS Association supports further research related to the use of cannabis for ALS but also issues a cautious approach to the use of marijuana as a drug of choice based on current evidence.

Crohn's Disease (CD)

It has long been known that cannabis has anti-inflammatory properties that are effective in bowel disorders. In ancient times, marijuana was smoked to get relief from abdominal pain, diarrhea, and cramping. Subjectively, patients with Crohn's disease have used cannabis for ages and reported a reduction in abdominal pain and cramping, diarrhea, and joint pain. Animal research done over more than ten years has decisively proved that cannabis and its various ingredients decrease gut inflammation. Crohn's disease is one of the very few diseases for which a human clinical trial has been done with cannabis to prove its efficacy. In this study, which was published in 2013, subjects were given inhaled marijuana twice daily for eight weeks. The trial concluded that cannabis can resolve symptoms of pain and nausea, improve appetite and sleep, has minimal side effects, and gives patients a break from steroid treatment that has serious side effects. However, the effects are short term, and after stopping it for two weeks, all symptoms may recur.

Whether it has disease-modifying properties has been debated, and no succinct evidence for progression or resolution currently exists. The exact mechanism of action involves its peripheral actions in the gut as well as centrally in the brain. Patients who smoke marijuana are much more likely to have had surgery for Crohn's disease. It is unclear if this means that smoking marijuana worsens the disease so that surgery is needed, or if sicker patients self-medicate to get relief from their symptoms.

Glaucoma

Glaucoma is a condition that threatens the vision because of optic nerve dysfunction resulting most commonly from high pressure within the eyes. Like the other conditions mentioned above, there is subjective description of reduction of intraocular pressure (IOP, pressure within the eye) in patients with glaucoma who smoked marijuana, because they responded partially or negligibly to standard treatments. Smoking marijuana reduces pressure within the eyes of all individuals, whether they suffer from glaucoma or not and may seem like a good treatment option. However, because of the required frequency of its use every three hours, the side effects are intolerable. They include sedation, dry mouth, dizziness, depression, confusion, weight gain, and so on. Smoke can cause damage to the lungs too when used in such high doses. It may be used as eye drops instead of inhalation but its penetration to reach inside the eye in proportions required for its effect is very small. And lastly, glaucoma is caused by optic-nerve dysfunction that can result from many reasons, with high IOP being only one cause. Marijuana has not been shown to have any effect on other possible causes of glaucoma such as blood supply to the optic nerve.

The American Glaucoma Society position statement on the use of marijuana for glaucoma is that "although marijuana can lower the IOP, its side effects and short duration of action, coupled with a lack of evidence that its use alters the course of glaucoma, preclude recommending this drug in any form for the treatment of glaucoma at the present time."

Cachexia/Wasting Syndrome

This is usually seen in patients with AIDS, cancer, or advanced dementia when they have very poor appetite and consistently lose weight with failure to thrive. Several small clinical trials have demonstrated that marijuana in inhaled or oral form stimulates appetite, stops weight loss, causes weight gain, and reduces nausea more than a placebo. These effects were found to be long term. Based on this moderate evidence for marijuana, the Federal Drug Association (FDA) had approved the use of dronabinol (synthetic form of cannabis, trade name Marinol) for use in AIDS patients with weight loss. It is well tolerated usually and has few side effects.

Severe Nausea and Vomiting

Dronabinol and nabilone are two synthetic forms of cannabis that are used for intractable chemotherapy-related nausea and vomiting. Dronabinol is FDA approved for this indication. According to the American Society of Clinical Oncology; however, it should not be used as a first-line treatment in this situation. There are excerpts of patients requesting that their doctors let them smoke marijuana to control nausea and doctors *not* disapproving it. Side effects as usual are a concern.

Posttraumatic Stress Disorder (PTSD)

Many patients with PTSD smoke marijuana to improve their sleep, appetite, and depression. The pattern of the use of marijuana in PTSD patients is somewhat different. Its use as a coping mechanism raises the risk for problematic addiction far more than usual, primarily because of heavier use leading to dependence. The motives for marijuana use in PTSD have been studied and results have revealed that mostly it is used for sleep, and in such cases, the frequency of use is much higher. Research also suggests that one of the cannabinoid chemicals may block negative memories or fear associated with the trauma in a process called *reconsolidation blockage*. Memories that remain latent and get reawakened need to be stabilized again for them to persist—a process called reconsolidation. If reconsolidation is blocked, then there is a weakening of the original memory. A single small study with PTSD patients who have nightmares showed that there was a reduction in those who used synthetic cannabis. These and other studies have prompted neuropsychologists to review the use of cannabis as a serious treatment for PTSD. In the United States, it has been approved in five states for use in PTSD. However, as in other conditions, a clinical trial would best prove the efficacy of marijuana in PTSD.

Movement Disorders

It has been stated that marijuana has neuroprotective characteristics that may help ameliorate some of the symptoms of movement disorders like Parkinson's disease or Huntington's disease. There may be a slight improvement in the quality of life and feeling of well-being in a subset of Parkinson's disease patients who have no dementia or psychiatric problems. It may help reduce tics but there are no benefits in tremors in MS or other types of complex movement disorders. No large clinical trials have been reported though several are currently ongoing, especially with Sativex spray. In short, cannabis is still not considered seriously for treatment of these conditions though random case reports may be seen.

Alzheimer's Dementia

The increasing incidence of dementia globally has encouraged researchers to find treatments that may stall or reverse the memory loss and cognitive impairment associated with different types of dementia. However, we lack medications that are clinically effective in dementia. Many clinicians have considered cannabinoids as a potential therapeutic approach to see if the various chemicals in cannabis may be of use. It is possible that cannabis may reduce the behavioral disturbances seen in dementia. Unfortunately, other than anecdotal descriptions, no scientific evidence exists that indicates that marijuana may be beneficial in dementia.

When I asked Joel Stanley about the challenges in marijuana-related research, he sketched a gloomy picture rife with a mental malaise against the very concept of medical marijuana that is impossible to break through. The state of Colorado examined their legacy in high cannabidiol (CBD) marijuana and approved millions of dollars in funding for research, none of which went to the Stanley Brothers because of archaic laws. Stringent federal regulatory policies that are arduous and grueling continue to prohibit research nationwide. I asked Joel how he would like to see the medical community engage with medical marijuana, and he had a one-point schema for us: advocate actively for marijuana research before it has a natural demise because of a lack of sustained support. Health-care providers carry considerable clout as a group and have the ability to bring about reform in health care effectively. The problem that I see is the controversial nature of the drug in question that polarizes health-care providers. Many physicians feel strongly about dismissing marijuana as nothing but dope and are rightfully concerned about the message we send to children and young adults. Others agree with decriminalizing marijuana but not legalizing it as a recreational drug. Skeptics also tag it as a gateway drug and claim that though it may be a relatively harmless controlled substance by itself, it encourages users to venture into the more serious world of hard drugs like cocaine and heroin.

As time passes, and I watch my parents, in-laws, aunts, and uncles grow older, it seems apparent that among them, they have a conundrum of disorders that may respond favorably to marijuana—progressive dementia, Parkinson's disease, crippling arthritis, chronic back pain, insomnia, seizure disorder, and so on. Some of them are on a cocktail of several heavy-duty medications that have many side effects like sedation and dizziness. I believe that a cannabis product could help either reduce the dosage or replace some of them, thus also alleviating side effects. It is possible that their quality of life could be improved considerably with a noninhaled form of marijuana, though there is no possible way for me to legally test this hypothesis in India.

It may seem unethical to discuss the use of a recreational drug for elderly family members, perhaps even criminal. But the point that I am trying to make is that even on a personal level, my conviction about marijuana is strong. I am also acutely aware that acceptance will not be easy and take a long time with many challenges to overcome. One of the first steps that must be taken is decriminalization for possession and use. Though the United States has less than 5 percent of the world's population, we have almost 25 percent of the total number of prisoners, a peculiar irony in the "land of freedom." The world looks upon America as a country that loves to jail its citizens. A significant proportion of these prisoners are held for possession and use of drugs like marijuana. These people languish in jail for what is inherently a minor offence and stretch the already overcrowded, poorly funded prison systems. It is well known that incarceration has an incredibly deleterious effect on the individual, his or her family, and society in general. Medical care during imprisonment and after release is compromised largely with poor transition-of-care programs in place. Health insurance gets complicated, often with discontinuation upon imprisonment, without automatic reinstatement on release.

Imprisonment for wrongful convictions of the innocent is not uncommon. This is even more harmful and has long-standing repercussions. Though crime in the United States has been decreasing slowly over the years, imprisonment of certain ethnic groups is high and rising, for example among African American men. The American criminal justice system needs serious overhauling for what has often been described as a monumental failure of the prison system for many reasons: one of which is related to marijuana and the other to wrongful convictions. Advocacy groups claim that minorities are unfairly targeted, mostly for petty crimes like marijuana possession, to keep certain numbers high that are used to measure the success of law enforcement in our society. It has been suggested that it is easier to target minorities that unfortunately could result in wrongful convictions. When justice fails, we fail too. Mr. Boyd is a prime example of that, as you will read in the next chapter.

CHAPTER 9
WHEN JUSTICE FAILS

"Yes, Doc, I was in prison for thirty years for a crime I did not commit, like any other black man in America," said Mr. Boyd as he lay back on his hospital bed.

It was early afternoon, and I was checking in on him to see how he was doing, though I had seen him earlier during morning rounds with my team of residents and medical students. In fact, I wanted to confirm what one of the residents had told me that day—he was wrongfully convicted when he was young and spent most of his youth incarcerated. It was a sickening story that I had a hard time believing. I had to confirm the truth behind it myself.

Mr. Boyd was a seventy-year-old, African American man with multiple, complex, medical problems for which he had a prolonged hospital stay that eventually took his life. We inherited him from another medical team at the month-end change of clinical rotation after he had already spent a couple of weeks in-house without any signs of improvement. I visited him at least twice a day, sometimes more. He had good days when things remained stable and bad days when he was worse. Lately, he had more bad days than good. He lived alone and did not have any family members who lived close by. He never had any visitors in the hospital.

"Mr. Boyd, how did that happen?" I tried to sound as discreet as I could amid nervous thoughts of maintaining professional propriety. Though doctors are trained to elicit a comprehensive medical history from patients, we also know when not to be intrusive. We almost never cross the fine line between professional history taking and being nosy. Right from the outset, medical students learn what *not* to ask. But sometimes the rapport we share with our patients makes it acceptable to informally chat with them about their lives. In fact, most patients like their doctors asking them personal questions about their family and so forth. It shows that they care and helps to shape a special connection, the most important piece of the doctor-patient relationship, in my opinion.

"Yes, Doc, it happens to black folks all the time. I was at the wrong place at the wrong time."

I couldn't bring myself to ask him the alleged crime that he got incarcerated for. Thirty years meant it was probably a grave one, like murder or child sexual assault. Feeling instant overpowering guilt, as if I had something to do with his misfortune, I just stood by his bed, transfixed, physically weak, acutely aware of my shallow breathing, crushing the urge to say something in sympathy. Even if I had tried to, I couldn't have got a word out without making my distress apparent to him. Doctors don't do that. We are hardwired to be strong professionals who should generally not demonstrate emotion unless it's a happy one. Besides, what could anyone have said that didn't sound hollow and superficial? During the time that we had spent together in the hospital, he was always cheerful and optimistic. Now I knew why. Being horribly sick was a breeze compared to being imprisoned for three decades for a crime committed by someone else. I had seen it on television once—a black man was exonerated and paid $750,000 in restitution. Mr. Boyd never got a single penny. Picture one day in prison for a crime you did not commit. Imagine *thirty years* living with that truth yet unable to prove your innocence.

I was once asked what makes me an authority on prisoners and the prison system in America. My answer was succinct—I am not one. But all it takes is kindness and humanity to understand the story above. As an employee of the Cook County Hospital and Health System for seven years in Chicago, I had the unique opportunity to take care of prisoners from the Cook County Jail, both inpatient and outpatient. There was a specific protocol for these prisoners and their guards for tight security. On admission, they were housed in one particular unit of the hospital and always had their shackles on, sometimes to the extent that the shackles cut through their skin. Police officers often sat together and chatted outside their rooms. The stories of the inmates were disturbing in many ways—for the gravity of their crimes, the sacrifices their families had to make, the remorse they felt, and their current medical illness. It was an exceptional experience that gave me insight into the unique barriers that we can come across in caring for prisoners in resource-limited conditions. I was encouraged to collaborate with pioneers in correctional medicine from across the country to publish a special themed edition of the monthly newsletter from the Society of General Internal Medicine with articles focusing on these challenges. Mr. Boyd has been one of the most touching life stories that I have ever come across.

It has been well documented that crime and incarceration rates are historically high among blacks. The literature is replete with reports of high imprisonment rates for men from poor black neighborhoods that gravely affect the families and communities. The imprisonment rate is defined as the number of prisoners under state or federal jurisdiction sentenced to more than one year per one hundred thousand US residents of all ages in a given year. In December 2012, imprisonment rates based on race and ethnicity revealed that 2.8 percent of black, 1.2 percent of Hispanic, and 0.5 percent of white males were in state or federal prison. In 2013, the US Department of Justice described trends of state prisoner admissions and releases between 1991 and 2011. There has been a decline in the year-end prison population every year since 2009 because of an increase in releases compared to admissions. In 2012, the prisoner population at year-end was 1.57 million compared to 1.59 million in 2011.

However, there has been an increase in new court commitments for violent offenses by blacks during this period, from 41 percent in 2001 to 47 percent in 2011. In 2011, 25 percent of all new white offenders, 34 percent of black offenders, and 36 percent of Hispanic offenders were sentenced for violent crimes. For blacks, this was an increase since 2006 when less than 30 percent of new admissions were for violent crimes. New admissions for murder and nonnegligent manslaughter between 2001 and 2011 showed a similar pattern with a reduction in whites from 29 percent to 24 percent and an increase in blacks from 46 percent to 51 percent.

Compared to white men, black men are six times more likely to be imprisoned, and the imprisonment rates for black men are at least four times those of white men in different age groups. For black men younger than age thirty-nine, the imprisonment rate is six times greater than that for white men of the same age. The biggest disparity is seen in male inmates aged eighteen to nineteen: black men in this age group were 9.5 times more likely to be in prison than white men of the same age. Black women aged eighteen to nineteen were three times more likely to be imprisoned than white women. Could this disparity be because of innocent African Americans who were wrongly convicted?

Historically, high numbers of young African-American men are spending their emerging adulthood in prison. In 2000, Arnett defined emerging adulthood as the period between age eighteen and twenty-five that defines the individual's foundation for adult life based on choices made in social, occupational, and behavioral domains. Exposure to prison restricts the complete development of the individual with subsequent failure to thrive as a productive member of society. High prevalence of parental imprisonment among blacks is a distinct childhood risk factor for crime and subsequent incarceration, thus feeding a vicious cycle that condemns an already susceptible population to inequality from one generation to the next.

"I'm so sorry for what happened to you, Mr. Boyd," I said feebly. Having spent most of his youth imprisoned, he never got married or had children. He had a low literacy level, few skills for gainful employment, and fragmented access to health care for most of his life. That is, until his health disabled him, and he was able to get disability benefits, which were meager at best. A whole life lost in one stroke of bad luck. The real criminal was never caught. It was someone he knew.

I have never been inside a prison. The only visuals I have seen are those on television and in films. Tim Robbins managed to escape after seventeen years of incarceration for crimes he denied in the movie *Shawshank Redemption*. In another Indian movie called *Veer Zaara*, a young Indian man was charged with being a spy and imprisoned for life in Pakistan without evidence. A female Pakistani lawyer finally fought for his release successfully and he returned home as a free man after languishing in prison for more than two decades. Both of these films were highly acclaimed for their story lines. Mr. Boyd neither escaped nor was he rescued. Images of Tim Robbins in the movie flitted in my mind. The brutal assaults, sexual violence, solitary confinement, all felt stomach-churningly real. I don't know if Mr. Boyd was subjected to violence during his incarceration. I did not want to know.

In a recent study that examined false conviction rates for criminal defendants on death row, it was estimated that at least 4.1 percent of them were innocent. The principal author of the paper is the editor and cofounder of the *National Registry of Exonerations*, a joint project between the University of Michigan and Northwestern University law schools. The registry has tracked wrongful convictions since 1989. According to this registry, most false convictions do not result in exonerations. As of April 2014, this registry had 1,326 exonerations with a record number of eighty-seven in 2013. California (119), Texas (114), and Illinois (112) had the highest exoneration numbers. The average time spent by the exonerees in prison was ten years, and the majority spent at least five to ten years in prison. Factors contributing to these convictions included perjury or false accusation, official misconduct, mistaken identification, misleading forensic evidence, and false confessions. A study of the basic patterns revealed that of all innocent prisoners, 92 percent were men and 46 percent were black. In every category except child sexual abuse—including sexual assault, homicide, and other crimes—more blacks were exonerated than others.

In a country where African Americans comprise only 15 percent of the total population, almost half of the wrongfully convicted prisoners were black.

"I am glad it's over, Mr. Boyd," I said.

Glad did not describe what my team felt for him. A few days later, he passed away silently, just as he had lived. The whole team wept for days. So many had failed him—law enforcement, the judiciary, health-care providers, and society in general. I couldn't help but go on a "what if" spree. What if he was not at the crime scene? What if the police had caught the real criminal? What if the courts had found him innocent in the beginning? What if he was found innocent during his protracted incarceration? What if he had a college education? What if he had a full-time job with benefits? What if he had access to better health care? What if he had a wife and children? What if...Endless ponderings provoked despondency in me for a life seemingly ravaged by misfortune.

He was clearly not the lone victim. Who can forget the mind-numbing details of the extreme torture inflicted on more than one hundred African American prisoners by Chicago Police Commander Jon Burge and his officers? Between 1972 and 1991, prisoners were systematically tortured with electric shock and suffocation to obtain coerced confessions leading to wrongful convictions. Andrew Wilson, an African American prisoner falsely accused of murder, sustained serious injuries after the torture and was examined by Dr. John Raba, the medical director of Cook County Jail. The extent of the injuries and Wilson's claim of innocence convinced Dr. Raba to initiate an investigation with the assistance of then Police Superintendent Richard Breczek that triggered a series of events resulting in Burge's termination from the Chicago Police Department. What followed was a gruesome account of sustained savagery by a white police officer and his colleagues inflicted on black prisoners to coerce confessions from them for crimes they did not commit. Ten years later a state review that cost $17 million proved that these wrongdoings were true. It incensed the residents of Chicago but because of a statute of limitations that could not result in any action against him. A civil suit against Burge eventually led to conviction and imprisonment for four and a half years in 2011. Most of the torture survivors received no compensation or psychological counseling. Twenty remain in prison because of convictions based at least partly on their coerced confessions. A few were freed after languishing for decades in prison.

Historical injustices like these because of confessions obtained through violence have been reported for centuries. The Miranda rulings were a result of landmark decisions by the US Supreme Court in the early-twentieth century against the use of coerced confessions as evidence for conviction. Yet injustices against African American men and women continue unabated, and they have given rise to movements like Black Lives Matter. The release of another black prisoner, Glenn Ford (now deceased), after conviction by an all-white jury and thirty years on death row for a murder he did not commit, forced me to wonder how many more remain unfairly imprisoned. He remains the longest serving death-row inmate in American history, and he spent twenty-nine years, three months, and five days in solitary confinement at a Louisiana prison. He received twenty dollars for a bus ride home and nothing else. Many strongly believe that the trial was riddled with appalling constitutional violations.

How does the legal system respond when a misjudgment has been committed? I say "committed" because it is no less than a crime. If you dig deeper into these cases, you will find stunning degrees of caprice and malevolence, methodically intertwined with contemptuous disregard for justice, and a voracious desire to win at any cost. Cops, lawyers, judges, juries, and correctional personnel repeatedly demonstrate their inherent bigotry and irrational penchant to punish the black man without evidence beyond a reasonable doubt. What equitable punishment should be bestowed on those who are a part of these horrific crimes? More often than not, the perpetrators escape penalties and are rarely convicted of wrongfully sentencing innocent people. Scores of black men on death row in his penitentiary were executed during Ford's incarceration. Were they all guilty as charged? Do states and lawyers apologize for their misdemeanors? Is an apology enough? Is money enough? If we had a choice to be incarcerated for three decades and get millions of dollars on release, would we ever opt to trade our freedom?

The Center on Wrongful Convictions at Northwestern University has been a champion for justice in wrongful convictions and has raised public awareness through evidence-based depictions of the current situation. Its groundbreaking legal actions have resulted in moratorium on state executions, criminal-justice reform, expanded DNA testing, increased funding, international reform, and compensation for exonerated prisoners. Many challenges remain; however, including the need to expand electronically recorded interrogation procedures in all criminal cases, implement standard procedures to enhance correct identification of suspects by witnesses, restrict actions that cause suffering from a stigmatizing experience, provide appropriate legal services for all prisoners, and establish structured compensation plans for exonerees.

The Innocence Project is a national litigation and public-policy organization dedicated to preventing future injustice by exonerating wrongfully convicted individuals through reform of the criminal-justice system and use of DNA testing. So far, more than three hundred wrongful convictions have been overturned, and many more are anticipated. This has been described as a masterful legacy of data on wrongful convictions, yet it only represents the tip of the iceberg. Of these DNA exonerations, 63 percent of defendants were African Americans.

A wrongfully convicted black man founded Resurrection after Exoneration (RAE) to rehabilitate exonerated prisoners in rebuilding their lives after years in prison. The mission of this non-profit organization is to help transition these people into society by providing them help in education, employment, and personal life. Exonerees and long-term prisoners face constant harassment at the hands of law enforcement and have poor access to health care after their release. Often their records reflect their incarceration even if they were wrongfully convicted. Most of them lose their family and many suffer from posttraumatic stress disorder. They become ineligible for student loans and housing and at times cannot vote. Essentially, these people are reduced to nothing and can barely exist from day to day without assistance. Organizations like RAE provide support in several ways to facilitate their return to society and carve a path for them by reinforcing their residual skills or interests.

This is not enough. Their confinement often reduces these people to a state that can be merely vegetative. The injustice done to them is irrevocable and conclusive. We can never return the years wasted in captivity. In 1765, Sir William Blackstone, an English scholar, said that it is better that ten guilty persons escape than one innocent suffer. He is considered a pioneer in common law and 10:1 became the Blackstone ratio that is a core philosophy taught in law schools. Ben Franklin, a founding father of the United States, said that the ratio should be 100:1 instead. A few radical personalities have disagreed with it and reverted the ratio to 1:10—better that ten innocents be sentenced than one guilty escape, lest the guilty cause havoc again. Pol Pot, Bismarck, and Dick Cheney fall into the latter category. Pol Pot was responsible for the annihilation of more than 20 percent of the Cambodian population. Bismarck was an intimidating German leader who fought wars with his neighboring countries. Cheney spoke in relation to terrorists in America. Some would say that law enforcement in the United States follows that rule at times.

Thomas Jefferson wrote, "We hold these truths to be self-evident, that all men are created equal, that they are endowed by their Creator with certain unalienable Rights, that among these are Life, Liberty, and the pursuit of Happiness." It remains to be seen if the United States can truly claim to be a land of freedom and opportunity without discrimination based on color. The racial bias that tarnishes the criminal-justice system gets attention in only a handful of prominent convictions. Without a sustained multipronged effort from the public, I daresay such discrimination will persist. A wise lawyer once said, "It's a legal system, not a justice system."

But whom do we blame when it's not the justice system but the society that fails us?

CHAPTER 10
WHEN SOCIETY FAILS

I t was almost dawn in the labor room where I was one of two interns on duty in a small tribal town in India. The hospital was affiliated with my medical school, and it was considered a large public-health, safety-net system that catered mostly to the vulnerable population. As a newly minted trainee on call, I felt anxious at the often-overwhelming action within the confines of a dynamic ward. It got quieter at night, and we even managed a few hours of sleep sometimes. My fellow intern was on her break, and I was sitting with a couple of nurses, catching up on all the patients. I looked up from the admissions register and saw her hovering just inside the door, dressed in an old beige sari, no slippers on her feet, looking around timidly. She was middle aged and slender, and I could see that she was married—she wore a *bindi* on her forehead and had red vermillion in the parting of her hair. Going by her appearance, she was extremely poor. The nurse beckoned her to the desk and asked her a few questions for intake.

My attention was caught when she replied to why she was there. She was raped a few hours ago. Her story was chilling. She was sleeping in her home on the floor with her two children in the other room when she heard her husband come in late at night. Her home was a ramshackle, tiny structure made of mud without any electricity. Her husband was an alcoholic and was usually home at that hour. She fell asleep again and woke up when she found him on top of her trying to have sex. There was complete darkness, so she lay there until he was almost done when she realized that it was not her husband. She screamed and resisted but was forcefully held down and her mouth clamped until the act was complete. The stranger ran away before she could see who it was. She found her husband passed out near the front door with alcoholic breath. Her kids were still sleeping. She walked several miles, all the way to the hospital, in the semidarkness.

She is the only rape victim I have personally met in my career who sought care with me after the assault. We advised her on how to file a police report later that day. She had no idea who the rapist was. She could not even describe him, as it was too dark. Medically she was stable and had not sustained any injuries. There were no rape kits or protocol to follow to collect semen or vaginal swabs, as DNA testing was not done then. I had no training whatsoever on how to deal with rape victims. We did not have psychological counseling services in the derelict public-hospital system. There were no social workers to help her in case her husband and family ostracized her, as was most likely to happen. By the time we were done, it was morning, and she was discharged home.

Basically, we did nothing to help her.

This was twenty-three years ago. Things haven't changed much since then. We still pretty much do nothing for rape victims. The brutal gang rape and subsequent death of a young woman in 2012 in New Delhi, India, captured the attention of people worldwide. As we heard, read, and watched in growing horror, the vicious attack in the heart of the capital city brought to the forefront a problem that has escalated in the past few decades to become a shocking depiction of the current state of women in India and other developing nations across the world. The sinister event led to much soul-searching and an increase in social consciousness that is unusual for a country of immense contradictions. While the political power in India rests with women leaders of different electoral groups in the capital and many states, the middle and lower socioeconomic classes exist in a primarily patriarchal society. This contrast in culture is prevalent in other regions of the subcontinent, Asia, and Africa. Sexual violence against women is common and is disregarded or hushed because of the social stigma that it brings. Rape victims face excessive hurdles at every stage, including filing a report with the often-hostile police, medical examination using the "two-finger" method, adequate legal help, and long, drawn-out, expensive, judicial processes. Unmarried women can be banished from their communities and lose all likelihood of getting married. It just seems easier to let go and disappear. Globally, sexual violence against women continues to be a serious human-rights and public-health problem, even in developed western countries like the United States.

As the travesty of the unfortunate Indian girl unraveled, the atrocities of Ariel Castro were discovered in the United States, a fifty-three-year-old man from Cleveland who held three women captive for more than a decade as his sex slaves. His story is a gruesome and sickening account of sustained sexual violence against women that borders on depraved bestiality.

As a trained Women's Health specialist and practitioner, the topic of sex crimes against women is of special interest to me. Sexual violence results in negative physical, mental, and psychosocial consequences that have a long-lasting impact on the victim as well as the family. The United Nations defines violence against women as "any act of gender-based violence that results in, or is likely to result in, physical, sexual, or mental harm or suffering to women, including threats of such acts, coercion, or arbitrary deprivation of liberty, whether occurring in public or in private life." In an in-depth review of global violence against women, *Lancet* published an article that describes the complex nature of the problem, which includes intimate-partner violence; sexual abuse by nonintimate partners; trafficking, forced prostitution, exploitation of labor, and debt bondage of women and girls; physical and sexual violence against prostitutes; sex-selective abortion, female infanticide, and the deliberate neglect of girls; and rape in war. In countries like India, sexual violence has been broadened to encompass other types of attacks on women including acid attacks, harassment, stalking, and "eve-teasing." According to Wikipedia, "Eve teasing is an euphemism used throughout South Asia, which includes (but is not limited to) India, Pakistan, Bangladesh, and Nepal for public sexual harassment or molestation (often known as "street harassment") of women by men, where the name "Eve" alludes to the very first woman, according to the biblical creation story." It's a common experience among women in these countries, sometimes a daily occurrence.

The past two decades have seen a sharp increase in the reporting of such acts and constant media coverage but not necessarily an appropriate increase in prosecution and conviction. Legal procedures, including the collection of forensic evidence, and irregularities in the conduct of routine investigations usually affect the fair administration of justice. Five south Asian countries (Bangladesh, India, Nepal, Pakistan, and Sri Lanka) have several gender-sensitive policies that are measurable by indicators that contribute to health. However, the mere presence of such policies is inadequate to realize true gender equity or empowerment of women and large inequities in women's health outcomes persist as a result. Since the death of the Indian girl, three years have passed, and the culprits have still not been sentenced.

In a not-so-surprising analysis from South Sudan, the world's newest nation, 82 percent of women and 81 percent of men agreed that women should tolerate violence to keep the family together. Even more worrisome was the finding that more women than men (47 percent vs. 37 percent) agreed that it was acceptable for men to beat their wives for sex. The authors used a Gender-Equitable Men scale to capture the perceptions of men in regard to the roles of both genders in family, domestic, and sexual life. They defined a gender-equitable man as one "who is respectful to women, who believes that men and women should have equal rights, who shares responsibility in the household," and is thus opposed to violence against women. This acquiescence of gender-biased practices is pervasive in many other countries. The literature is replete with case reports, narrative reviews, and cohort and longitudinal studies that chronicle the existence of these practices in all parts of the world, including the so-called developed nations where women are presumed to be more emancipated and independent.

It is well established that sexual assault victims have a higher prevalence of hypertension, obesity, dyslipidemia, heart disease, stroke, and negative lifestyle choices, like smoking, which may be adaptive responses to violence. The global economic burden is estimated to be in the tens of billions. A majority of rapes are by intimate partners. Any report underestimates the true prevalence of intimate-partner violence since it is considered a taboo topic for women in traditional patriarchal societies. Marital rape is unrecognized as a crime and women are expected to suffer through it as a necessary evil of society. Additionally, there is substantial evidence of violence outside the home, as in the case of child predators and women veterans. In fact, military sexual trauma is a well-recognized psychiatric disorder that results from sexual assaults during service and is known to cause depression, posttraumatic stress disorder, and alcohol abuse. In a recent study from Bangladesh, the authors opined that sexual harassment results in negative psychological impacts on adolescent girls, including loss of self-esteem and persistent feelings of insecurity. It is also well established that violent exposures are associated with depressive symptoms in women, including postpartum depression and increased under-five child mortality.

Screening for sexual violence is not a routine practice in primary care, and no guidelines by peer institutions like the United States Preventive Services Task Force have emerged to establish such a practice. Health-care providers and practices are ill equipped to help victims. Apart from nongovernmental organizations that may be able to help on a short-term basis, there remains a dearth of programs that address the proper rehabilitation of victims of sexual assaults. Preventing sexual assaults is even more critical. The problem has to be addressed on many different levels: political, legislative, judicial, social, medical, and personal. Emancipation of women remains fundamental, but a more crucial factor is a change in social attitudes toward women. For example, India has seen tremendous financial independence of women based on its commitment to the education of girls, but by itself this has not led to an increase in safety. In fact, it may have contributed to the problem, as women travel alone between school, college, and work at all hours of the day, thus exposing themselves to risks of attacks in a culture holding on fiercely to its patriarchal underpinnings. After the gang-rape incident, there were changes in rape laws in India. Laws related to sexual crimes were reassessed, and the very definition of rape was extended. However, marital rape was still not recognized, and army personnel remain immune to prosecution for sex crimes. It remains to be seen if stricter laws result in a reduction of crimes against women.

What has changed in India then since the Delhi gang rape? Some would say nothing and would not be wrong. Others remind us that we have indeed made progress. Sexual-violence incidents are reported more frequently now with perhaps a marginal improvement in assistance to victims in the reporting process. The powerful Indian media increasingly crusades for the victims, and widely telecast discussions on rape have created a more comfortable space for the conservative society to indulge in open debates. The intense stigma associated with rape is eroding, a definite sign of progress. Prosecution of culprits is on the rise and though trials are long drawn out with few sentences. Having said that, the sum total of all changes is only slightly above zero, and we still have a long way to go to improve the safety of women in our society.

In the United States, sexual-violence data are equally horrific. According to the CDC, one in five women was raped at some time in her life, and almost half were younger than eighteen years of age. One in ten high-school girls was forced to have sexual intercourse. More than ten thousand women were treated in emergency rooms for injuries from sexual assault between 2004 and 2006, and more than thirty-two thousand pregnancies result from rape every year. Apart from the physical, mental, and psychosocial impacts, the economic toll of intimate-partner violence against women was documented in 2003 to cost the United States approximately $8.3 billion. Those who were assaulted as a child are unfortunately more likely to report further assaults as adults. Sexual violence against boys and men has been on the rise too. There is scant data about it and sporadic incidents are plenty. Sexual-assault incidents in prisons are well documented. However, stringent laws and rigorous punishment for culprits are better in the United States than in Asian and African countries where a large majority either go unreported or infrequently result in a conviction.

No doubt, we need to do more for women across the world. However, the focus must be on pertinent issues that matter the most to empower them. In my opinion, access to health care, education, safety, jobs, and childcare are five of the most pressing needs of today's women. Spending a hundred million dollars to investigate a questionable drug that could stimulate sexual desire in women is not an urgent need. The recent commotion created by the "pink Viagra" garnered tremendous debate in medical and nonmedical circles. It seems incredibly strange that when women are besieged by real problems that affect basic existence, pharmaceutical investigators opted to spend their time, energy, and dollars on a condition that is not even a disorder. Is the pink pill a tool of female empowerment? Or is it just another absurd attempt to commercialize one more issue related to women in a cacophonous incongruity that clashes with the core principles of women's health?

CHAPTER 11

PINK, BUT NOT ROSY

What is hypoactive sexual desire disorder (HSDD) in women? Is it a disease? Is it scientifically proven that having low libido in women is a disorder? When was it classified as a medical condition? Do women need to *feel* sick for a diagnosis? Is it just all in her head? Is it a psychological or mental disorder? How do we make comparisons without defining what the normal sexual-desire level in women is?

Or is it just a marketing strategy by the big bad wolf, Big Pharma, to prepare for brisk business prior to the release of flibanserin, the female equivalent of Viagra?

In a recent study published in an international ethics journal co-owned by the *British Medical Journal*, the authors concluded that HSDD is an imaginary condition that was invented as a marketing ploy to sell flibanserin, or the "pink Viagra." An investigational drug at the time of writing, it was being studied as a treatment for low sexual desire in premenopausal women. Another writer called it an "utterly hallucinatory invention." When I initially read the articles, my first reaction was of immense indignation.

How dare they? The investigators must all be men. How typical of the medical community that has chosen to entirely focus on male sexual disorders and been almost flippant about female sexual dysfunction. Not only was I offended as a middle-aged woman but I was also concerned about the implications of the report as a medical specialist in women's health, who has given many a talk on, as well as treated patients "supposedly" with HSDD. But then it made me think a little more profoundly about HSDD. I don't remember studying about it in medical school or during residency. As a junior faculty in an academic hospital, I never heard my mentors in the Section of Women's Health discuss it. It was only a few years ago when we were presenting a talk on "sexual disorders in women" that I came across HSDD. It was right around the time that clinical trials with flibanserin were ongoing. A PubMed literature search revealed the same—HSDD came into existence when flibanserin was "discovered."

The thought made me virtually stop in my tracks. A made-up disease? I had never heard of anything like that. How can anyone make up diseases? Medicine is a science and the body suffers from disorders that are well recognized and documented. But curiosity and a dreadful feeling led me to surf the web and to a whole new world of "disease mongering" or "condition branding," a not un-common practice by powerful pharmaceuticals intent on selling new drugs for disorders hitherto unrecognized. In 2010, flibanserin was being studied as an antidepressant. Though it was found to be ineffective in relieving depression, a few women experienced a slight increase in sexual desire during the clinical trial. This alleg-edly spurred the pharmaceutical industry and involved scientists to "invent" HSDD. Other conditions that have apparently been de-scribed to be a result of disease mongering include restless leg syn-drome, gastroesophageal reflux disease, irritable bowel syndrome, premenstrual dysphoric disorder, and so on.

I was shocked. Physicians like me have believed these disease entities to be legitimate disorders that have specific drugs available for treatment. That they could be "pseudo disorders" inherently discovered to sell drugs is like a slap in the face of clinicians across the world. I feet bitter and resentful for having fallen into the trap for so many years. Prozac received a new, more feminine-sounding name, Sarafem, and it was sold as an effective medication to young women for "premenstrual dysphoric disorder." I have prescribed it myself to many women who complained of feeling irritable during the days preceding menstruation. But now that I think about it, why is it considered a sickness to have mood variations related to normal, cyclic hormonal changes? Women have had these symptoms since the day they were created. It is a normal part of their physiology. It may not be pleasant, but is it a disorder? The level of deceit is outrageous and shocking to the core. With HSDD, I am determined to let the truth out, and here it is.

HSDD has been defined in the *Diagnostic and Statistical Manual of Mental Disorders*, fifth edition (*DSM-5*), as persistent or recurrent deficiency (or absence) of sexual fantasies or thoughts, and/or desire for or receptivity to sexual activity, which causes personal distress. A feeling of distress associated with it is a necessary component for diagnosis. Many women have low libido but do not necessarily worry about it or experience distress because of it. I have had countless patients in my clinical practice across the world who either practice abstinence or indulge in sex only for their partner's sake with negligible desire.

Take the case of Martha, my forty-five-year-old patient who was married twice and had three children. She was starting to experience a few symptoms that I suspected were related to perimenopause, like hot flashes, mild mood swings, and irregular menses. When I asked her about vaginal dryness or discomfort during sex, another symptom of perimenopausal women, she shrugged dismissively and said, "Meh." I asked her what she meant by that. She looked away and mumbled that she was never "into sex" anyway, so she had not noticed anything different. As we talked more, I found out that she had almost never had a pleasurable experience during sex but considered it her "duty" to indulge in intercourse to keep the men in her life happy. Neither the lack of a libido nor satisfactory sexual events seemed to bother her. She further said she considered it normal for all women to feel this way. In her sporadic and fleeting conversations with her friends and family members, she perceived other women to be in a similar state as her.

I felt a little alarmed after I had this discussion with Martha, and I am inclined to reassure women that this is not true. Women should normally have a healthy level of sexual desire and indulge in sexual activities that are satisfactory. Though almost half of women (40 percent) may experience low sexual desire, distress is reported in approximately 10–15 percent of women, categorizing them as having HSDD. Men suffer from HSDD too but the prevalence rate is less than half in women and is more straightforward. It has been touted as the most common female sexual disorder, which also includes other problems like female orgasmic disorder, sexual aversion disorder, sexual arousal disorder, and sexual pain disorder. Underlying physical, psychological, and social issues have been reported as causative factors, and nonpharmacologic treatment includes education, counseling, and psychotherapy. Non-FDA-approved drugs are occasionally used off label, including bupropion, testosterone, and estrogen. Osphena (ospemifene) is widely advertised on television and is a selective, estrogen-receptor modulator like tamoxifen that improves the integrity of vaginal and vulvar linings and relieves pain during intercourse. However, at the time of this writing, the FDA had just approved flibanserin for hypoactive sexual desire in a controversial move that is widely believed to be influenced by pressure from the feminist brigade.

There is considerable criticism of how HSDD became a "psychiatric" disorder with its own *DSM-V* definition. It has been suggested that much of the research was conducted by the pharmaceutical industry in anticipation of selling a drug that could potentially tap a $2 billion market. The concept that having a low libido makes a woman sick when she may not feel sick is by itself a contentious statement. Women often consider various difficult-to-measure components of a healthy sexual life as critical, including a strong emotional component with an empathetic and compassionate relationship with men. In the absence of such a relationship, women may not have the desire to indulge in sexual activity. Does this make them sick? Or does it merely result in unnecessary pressure on women to "think" that they are sick and need medical treatment? Can we safely say that the presence of such a medication in the market will not increase the demands on women from their partners in an all-pervasive environment that is already tilted against women because of widespread sexual abuse? The very premise that low libido in women is a product of a chemical imbalance in the brain is highly debatable. Is it on par with disorders like schizophrenia, bipolar disease, and major depression, genuine mental disorders resulting from chemical imbalances? Would it be effective in women in abusive relationships or victims of intimate-partner violence? Could it potentially escalate the degree of abuse?

Studies with flibanserin define a "desire day" for women as one in which the sexual desire is more than "no desire." This definition confuses me. How do we measure or quantify the degree of desire in women? Is it 1 percent more or 55 percent more or 100 percent more than "no desire"? Is the "range" of sexual desire the same in all women? Is desire different from excitement, or are they the same? In men, the desire should be enough to result in penile erection that will hopefully end in ejaculation, thus making it simple to quantify desire. Any desire that results in less than these end points will be contained within the definition of erectile dysfunction; this is a desire, which does not result in penile erection and ejaculation. For women, there are no such valid end points other than an orgasm that can capture a woman's sexual response and determining that a drug like flibanserin is effective in enhancing sexual desire based on an intangible scale that differs from woman to woman seems puzzling to me. How do we really know or compare desire in different women? Even more perplexing is the assumption that the presence of any degree of sexual desire, no matter how miniscule, is an indication that the drug is effective—even if the enhanced desire does not always end in a satisfactory sexual event. How does this change the sexual health of women in a positive way? Are women supposed to be happy with just an enhancement of sexual desire? The ambiguous "desire score" is a self-reported value, much like the "pain scale." Universally, physicians like me use the pain scale from one to ten for our patients (ten being the worst) to try to gauge the degree of pain that the patient is suffering from, knowing precisely that this is the most unscientific method of history taking. In spite of this, we prominently display laminated pain scales with a sad smiley face at one and an agonized face at ten in all areas of a hospital or clinic that are accessed by patients! Is the desire score as unscientific as the pain scale? Daily diaries have not been proven to be the most systematic way of assessing sexual response in women in a meaningful way. Most studies done with flibanserin rely heavily on these self-reported diaries. No wonder the FDA was unconvinced about the efficacy of the drug the first two times. As an aside, I am amused by the names of the studies done with flibanserin— most of them are named after flowers! It's an obvious attempt to label the female variety of *homo sapiens* as delicate flora that needs protection and nurturing. Or is it just a patriarchal take on the proverbial weaker gender that is historically believed to wilt at the slightest harshness?

Of all the discussions about flibanserin that I read and heard about, the one that I found the most amusing was its description as a drug that sparks a woman's desire by "fiddling with her brain chemicals." Really now? Many women would agree that the brain chemicals are not the body part that needs fiddling with to arouse them! Others would concur and say it's all in the "head" for a woman! Thus, we remain clueless about what women really want. One of the main reasons why the medical community has not been able to find a solution to female sexual disorders is because female sexuality is a lot more complex than male sexuality. In the clinical trials done with flibanserin and other related drugs that compared the drug to a placebo and analyzed their efficacy in enhancing sexual desire and experiences, the placebo group showed a significant improvement too. How do we explain that? The difference between the two groups (one who took the drug, the other who took a placebo) is pretty unimpressive though statisticians will have you believe that it is "significant" in their world—0.8 more sexually satisfying events every month for those on the drug. Hallelujah! And we women are supposed to jump for joy and somersault in delight at this colossal shift in our sexual lives? This just reminds me of a quote that has been variously accredited to Disraeli, Mark Twain, and an unknown person: "There are three kinds of untruths: lies, damned lies, and statistics." We know very well that what may be statistically significant does not always translate into a clinically meaningful outcome. So based on this rather flimsy evidence, we are poised to see a potential "revolution" in the sexual lives of women, at a mind-boggling cost that could have been used to bring happiness to women's lives in many other ways! Forgive me if I am underwhelmed.

I am also a little mystified about the cohort of women chosen for these drugs—premenopausal only. What about postmenopausal women who clinically have more problems related to sexual dysfunction because of hormonal changes? In the past, hormonal therapy like transdermal testosterone patches has shown some benefits in enhancing sexual desire and meaningful sexual activity in postmenopausal women. Even in these studies, the definitions of sexual desire are vague—for example, an increase was defined from "seldom" to "sometimes." I can almost hear feminists go ballistic—sometimes? Even nonfeminists would argue that it is desirable to experience a strong libido more often than just sometimes. By any means, this does not seem like a scientific way of measuring libido in women.

Some studies describe the use of validated tools like a sexual-activity log and a personal-distress scale, which are considered standard assessment tools by researchers in the field. However, until and unless researchers and health-care providers understand and classify sexual desire in women in a more scientific way, we will continue to be fooled by the pharmaceutical industry into thinking that we have a solution to a problem that is so poorly defined. Hard measures like quality of life and interpartner relationships are definitely more robust and translate into meaningful outcomes. After all, women complain more about their dissatisfaction with communication, passion, affection, and intimacy in their relationships with men than any genital-related behaviors—a fact scientifically proven that should be taken seriously when assessing female sexual disorders in a clinical setting.

I am seriously concerned about the trend of disease mongering or condition branding or pseudodiseases that the pharmaceutical industry has been accused of, because it has diverted the scientific community away from genuine regard for the underlying facts about low sexual desire in women and what women really want. I think that what women want is to be understood as a whole rather than a sum of the parts and ignoring or underestimating the impact of the nongenital component of a healthy sexual life in future research would be like putting a square peg in a round hole, no pun intended. Until then, it's advisable that women need not pump up their expectations and all of us prepare for mind-numbingly irritating advertising. Hey, I even asked my financial adviser if it would be smart to invest in the company making the drug. Unfortunately, it's not a public company yet, and my feeble attempt at cashing in on a health-care-related phenomenon that I think I am mildly entitled to, was an epic fail. A few days after the FDA approval, the company that spent $100 million to study flibanserin was bought for billions of dollars by larger fish in the big pharma sea.

Recently, I watched famous celebrity Jenny McCarthy on television talking about flibanserin. She said that after reading about it she realized that "it messes with your brain but doesn't give you a lady boner," How succinctly put it in simple words! Flibanserin is the fiddler on the roof! An unnecessary one, I believe. Instead of spending $100 million on a fancy drug that may give a handful of women a teeny enhancement of their sexual lives, how about we try to be nice to them? Respect, love, gentleness, and appropriate flirting will get us a better outcome than any brain messing. Thoughtful foreplay will fuel their desire additionally.

It will be a jolly day for women when a Viagra-like drug is released in the market that suitably addresses the multifaceted sex life of all women alike, pre- and postmenopausal, and yields happy endings just like in men. And then we will truly be able to sing along with Cindy Lauper—indeed, girls just wanna have fun too. For now, girls will continue to have fun just as before—merrily and in high heels!

CHAPTER 12
HEALING WITH HEELS

"Hi, Dr. Pandey. How are you?"

I looked up from my desk and saw Eboniqua standing just inside the door of my clinic room. Ebony, as she was fondly addressed, was an African American, male-to-female, transgender woman who worked as a peer educator at the HIV center where I had worked for several years. She was slimly built and almost six feet tall.

"Hey, Ebony! Good to see you."

I waved her into my room and turned around to look at her.

"You look different today."

I couldn't quite put my finger on what was different. Though Ebony was born a man, her attire was always somewhat over-the-top in a diva-inspired style, as if she was about to embark on a burlesque show. Animal prints, big hair, striking makeup, and of course—pointy, tall, slim, very high-heeled shoes that she teetered on. I never failed to be amazed at how she never slipped or fell and always seemed to have a tremendously confident walk.

"Aha, you are wearing flat shoes today!" I exclaimed. Indeed, I had never seen her in flats. She was five inches shorter and looked timider, almost demure.

"Yes, Doctor, I have back pain and my chiropractor told me it was from my heels. I came to ask you if this is possible. I cannot wear flat shoes every day!" she whimpered.

Now that was truly a problem. Flat shoes would definitely rain on her swag parade. In addition, her participation in drag events would be decimated. Who wants a drag queen without high heels?

High-heeled shoes have historically been very popular among women across the globe. Those who can wear them effortlessly are the envy of those who cannot. Though some women may scoff at such fashionable footwear, deep down most of us would love to slay a pair of stilettoes. Models on the catwalk strutting flawlessly up and down the ramp, their centers of gravity seemingly rock steady, often elicit gasps of admiration.

My research on high-heeled shoes and the health aspects of long-standing use led me to some interesting facts about them. In high fashion, there are three categories of heels: low heel, less than 2.5 inches high; mid heel, 2.5–3.5 inches high; and high heel, higher than 3.5 inches. Then there are heels for men, cowboy heels and Cuban heels—a special type of reinforced heels on a stocking, mostly created for men.

Men have been wearing heels for longer than women!

Historically, the concept of heels originated in the ninth century when male horseback warriors in Persia wore heeled boots and shoes that were designed to prevent the foot from sliding out of the stirrups when they were riding horses. These shoes were not a fashion item and were popular for their practical purpose. When the warriors stood up on the horse to shoot an arrow during battles, the square-heeled shoes secured them in a steady grip to allow a firm posture.

Try doing that on the pointy heels of modern-day shoes and risk a fall on your face!

In the sixteenth century, the Persian emperor, in an effort to seek allies against the Ottoman Empire, sent his diplomats to collaborate with the aristocrats of Europe. The heeled footwear of the Persians fascinated the Europeans and gradually became a popular fashion item among high-society men. The king of France, Louis XIV, whose rule for almost three-quarters of a century is one of the longest monarchies in history, can be seen wearing his heels proudly and in full masculinity in paintings from that era. That those heels were more like "blocks" and quite ugly is pretty evident. These fashion-deprived accessories would make contemporary women balk!

Soon European women were lured to wear high heels too. By the eighteenth century, men had stopped wearing them, and during the French Revolution, high heels disappeared for a brief period. But by the mid-nineteenth century, high heels returned and were quite the rage among women, becoming increasingly accepted as a critical aspect of female sexuality. Initially, women in pornography were the only ones to wear them, as they were not built for walking even moderate distances but could be worn in photographs. Later, more practical and creative designs emerged that became popular among all women.

This gender-bending history of high heels is the premise of where we are today—high heels have become an important fashion accessory, ubiquitously found in the closets of women. Who can forget the three thousand pairs of shoes, many of them high heeled, that were discovered in the home of Imelda Marcos, the first lady of Philippines? According to a recent survey by the American Podiatric Medical Association, half the women surveyed wore high heels. The average number of heels owned by heel-wearing women was nine, though almost half the time they rarely wore them.

"Yes, it's possible, Ebony. Back pain is a common problem in those who wear high heels for prolonged periods of time." I gave her an honest answer.

The disappointed look on her face prompted me to ask her a few more questions.

"How many hours a day do you wear heels?"

"Well, it all depends. I prefer to wear them whenever I am out of my home. Sometimes when I have visitors I wear them at home too."

"How high are your heels usually?" I asked.

"At least four inches. I prefer five inches, though. It makes me feel sassy." She did a mini twirl as she spoke.

My next question was one that I sort of knew the answer to, being a woman who likes heels.

"Why do you wear heels?"

She pondered for a moment.

"I like how it makes me feel, more feminine, more ladylike."

I don't know who invented high heels, but all women owe him a lot.

—Marilyn Monroe

So why do women wear high heels?

Almost entirely because of cosmetic reasons, some would say. It gives them height and slenderness, makes legs look longer, and enhances the gait, overall adding to the seductiveness with a sleek, svelte look. Shorter women can reach higher up that gives them a practical purpose.

A few women claim that they cannot wear flat shoes because of problems with their feet, especially the arches, that compels them to wear heels. Even a few months of wearing high heels can cause a shortening of the Achilles tendon and calf muscles so that when women switch to flats or flip-flops, it causes pain and inflammation because of stretching leading to "flip-flop-itis." Thus wearing heels becomes essential to avoid pain.

The business dress code for some professionals, such as lawyers, corporates, and bankers, includes heeled shoes for female employees as a compulsory requirement. The employer may fire an employee for not complying with such rules if it negatively affects the business as per a Supreme Court verdict in 2005, according to an article published in 2013 (J. Lorkowski, M. Mrzygłód, I. Kotela, E. Kiełbasiewicz-Lorkowska, and I.Teul, "Footwear according to the 'business dress code,' and the health condition of women's feet— computer-assisted holistic evaluation," *Annales Academiae Medicae*

Stetinensis 59, no. 2 [2013]: 118–28). This study examined the effect of high-heeled shoes in women at work and concluded that 70 percent of women suffered from foot pain and functional limitation. Several airlines require their women employees to wear heeled shoes when working. The Israeli airline El Al was recently in the news for changing their rules for female flight attendants who were required to wear high-heeled shoes until the flight took off whereas they could change into comfortable shoes once on board, though this could be dangerous in an emergency. It attracted considerable negative attention as male employees were exempt from such requirements.

Controversial evidence indicates that wearing heels helps tighten muscles of the pelvic floor and may reduce urinary incontinence. In 2008, Dr. Maria Cerruto, an Italian urologist and self-proclaimed patron of high heels, conducted a study that concluded that the downward flexion of the foot from wearing heels alters the posterior tilt of the pelvis that enhances the contractility of the pelvic-floor muscles. This could, at least theoretically, relax the muscles to reduce pelvic pain and improve incontinence of urine. The study was presented as a poster that was received enthusiastically and went on to win the best poster presentation at the European Association of Urology Conference.

I believe time wounds all heels.

—John Lennon

"There are other problems that you could have from wearing such high heels," I said.

"Really? Like what, Doctor?"

Evidently, there are quite a few. There is certainly a concern among health-care providers about problems caused exclusively by heels. Podiatrists, chiropractors, and orthopedic surgeons are the specialists who see a majority of such conditions. High heels redistribute the body weight and cause a change in the curvature of the body. A three-inch heel may tip the body forward by as much as ten to fifteen degrees and alter the center of gravity. Some of the common complaints include low-back pain, leg and foot pain, unsteady gait, knee and hip pain, as well as accidental injuries because of a misstep, slip, or fall.

Anatomical distortions that can cause pain and appear unaesthetic include hammertoes, bunions and corns, blisters, ingrown toenails, and abnormal spine curvatures. Warmth and moisture can cause athlete's foot and fungal infections of the nails. The knee joint can be overly stressed and lead to early degenerative changes and osteoarthritis. Similar changes can occur in other joints too, including hip, ankle, foot, and spine. Wearing heels may at least partly be responsible for the higher incidence in women of hip and knee osteoarthritis. Plantar fasciitis is a painful inflammation of the soft tissues of the sole of the feet, often caused by faulty footwear. Misalignment can cause poor posture and increase risk for falls and fractures. Tendon and ligament sprains are common. Consequently, the quality of life can be substantially reduced for those who suffer from the deleterious biomechanical effects of high heels. Interestingly, in a few studies, it has been disproved that wearing higher heels results in more foot problems. But the majority of studies have shown that high heels cause a stiffness of the Achilles tendon and shortening of the calf muscle, both of which can pathologically alter the gait as well as cause muscle fatigue and increase the risk for sprain. Poor venous circulation can cause aching in the legs and varicose veins.

Chronic, low-back pain is one of the commonest problems in the world and has a multitude of causes. It is well known that any anatomical abnormality in the lower extremities can be functionally problematic for the musculoskeletal unit of the lower back. Hyperpronation (extreme inward rotation of the foot that flattens the arch) has been linked to low-back pain and can be caused by wearing high heels for long periods. Often, this back pain can be alleviated by simple foot orthotics. Of course, saying good-bye to the heels becomes essential, no matter how painful it may be to let go of them!

Heeled footwear has been linked in a somewhat bizarre manner with a higher incidence of schizophrenia. In a study published in 2004, it was claimed that walking stimulated brain receptors that improve cognitive function. Those who wear high heels have an altered gait and thus a weaker stimulation of these receptors leading to a chemical imbalance predisposing to schizophrenia. The authors claimed that the global pattern of prevalence of schizophrenia indicates that in colder countries where flat shoes are more often worn, as well as in children who start walking in winter, there is a lower prevalence of schizophrenia. The study was criticized as unscientific and mostly dismissed by academic scholars.

"I am never going to stop wearing heels, come hell or high water! I will bear the pain instead," she said with a defiant look on her face.

"That's not a great idea," I tried to point out, though pretty common, I said to myself.

According to a 2014 American Podiatric Medical Association survey, 71 percent of women who wore heels experienced pain, but almost half of them could withstand wearing heels that were three inches high, even with pain. Moral of the story, women will continue to wear high-heeled shoes come "heel" or high weather! Ebony was one of them.

"Perhaps you could take some precautions," I said.

"That I am willing to consider."

I gave her a list of helpful tips to mitigate the damage from high heels. Wear the lowest heels that you can possibly, ideally not more than two inches (which I knew would be impossible for her when she was performing but recommended for the rest of the time). A leather insole would provide a better grip and prevent slips, whereas a heel lift has been shown to relieve low-back pain. The toe end should be as wide as possible. Pointed-toe shoes can cause deformities and bunions. Interestingly, a foot may be larger in size during the late afternoon and evening. It could be because of swelling from the hydrostatic pressure of standing and walking. Buying shoes later in the day ensures a better fit. Stretching exercises of the feet, toes, Achilles tendons, and leg muscles before putting on heels and after removing them will enhance the overall flexibility and strength. If possible, removing shoes intermittently for a few minutes every now and then may give relief from discomfort.

A tough set of rules for the hardened heel wearer!

Regardless, Ebony tried her best. She dropped her heel size a couple of inches, though never going below two inches—the mourning period was staggered, with a step-by-step reduction in heel size, no pun intended! Her back pain resolved, though she did have mild foot pain at times. She was happy to tolerate that.

I am embarrassed to confess that the day I wrote this chapter, I inadvertently went shopping and bought my first pair of three-inch peep-toe stilettoes! By the time I realized what I had done, it was too late—too late for regret, too late to return, too late to let go, too late to relinquish. I felt a little ashamed, not just by the hypocrisy of the situation but also the shallowness of my guilty pleasure. I know that I will be one of those women who will rarely wear them. I may even tolerate the pain for a short period when I do. And yes, I daresay that the thrill of feeling taller is incomparable to any other. One of my friends remarked, clearly in a bid to buttress my guilt, that it's never a good idea to follow your own advice. But what is crystal clear in this discussion about accessories that enhance outward beauty is that as humans, we are obsessed with the visual presented to us. It doesn't matter if we are men or women or transgender—we want to like what we see, and thus we strive to achieve that outward graphic pictorial to please ourselves and others. Who decided that tall is better than short, or more attractive? Why do we find flat shoes unappealing? They are comfortable, far more productive, and protect our feet. There are negligible health risks associated with them. Men in general almost always wear flat shoes and do not need to enhance their height falsely. If pretty is what appeals to us, we can find a wide variety of designs. But it leads us to the inevitable question—is beauty really in the eyes of the beholder? What is the rationale behind humans gravitating toward superficial appearances even when the pitfalls are obvious?

From wearing woven-hair extensions that itch and hurt, make-up that can cause allergic reactions, jewelry that may produce dermatitis, long acrylic nails that host harmful bacteria, painful tattoos, waxing, threading, and body piercings to uncomfortable body shapewear and high-heeled shoes, men and women strive to attain an outward appearance goal that is driven by personal preferences. Beliefs about beauty are disparate; the pursuit of physical perfection is universal. Is accepting our physical appearance in its natural state that difficult? What makes us try hard to be taller, fairer, darker, hairier, slimmer, than what we were born with? And even more thought provoking is why have we as a society made this type of behavior an appropriate and acceptable practice by setting standards of body image that are irrational?

Twenty-one years ago when I met my husband for the first time in a gathering arranged by our parents in India, I was told that the prospective groom was six feet four inches tall. I thought I packed quite a punch at five feet two inches. In an arranged marriage like ours, physical compatibility based on external appearance is a major criterion for a "good match." Height is critical. So is complexion. When I was getting ready to meet the family, I chose to wear flat shoes with my outfit. My mother was somewhat alarmed to see this and strongly recommended that I wear at least two-inch-heeled shoes; otherwise, a glaringly obvious mismatch might jinx the alliance. Though I was sympathetic toward her as an anxious Indian parent trying hard to "find" a well-matched groom for her child, I bluntly refused. I felt like the guy should know the truth about my short height and make a decision based on his choices. It obviously all worked out in the end, as we got married and are still together. Friends and family occasionally tease us with due respect, but the difference in our heights has never been a problem. Yet I have made a personal choice to usually wear heeled footwear, especially when we are together. It is inexplicable. I am sure my choice has nothing to do with the height of my spouse. Is it because of parental influence? I doubt it since my mother never wears heels. Perhaps it's the notion that five feet two inches is just not enough—five feet four inches is somehow better. Is it? I know that I feel happier in heels. Does altering our physical appearance to an accepted conventional societal standard always provide us with happiness? And if it does, should we be ostracized for it?

The stupendous success of the cosmetic and fashion industry as well as reconstructive surgery indicates that we want infallible flawless good looks at any cost. But when is enough, enough? Enough becomes too much when it affects physical or mental health negatively, as in the case of Ebony. The recent death of a Justin Bieber lookalike who spent more than $100,000 in facial-reconstructive surgery to resemble the star has raised questions about the dangers of addictive behaviors regarding physical appearances. We can never achieve perfection in our lives, because we don't know what perfection is. It is inherent within us, as human beings, to be dissatisfied with things. But as long as we remain fit and well balanced, it is acceptable to make small changes that may give us joy. Fashion is good for your soul. Make sure that it's good for your body too.

For Ebony, life was tough as a transgender woman. She got real happiness from only a handful of things—one of them was wearing high heels. She is one of a large group of people who struggle daily with their sexual identity at significant personal cost with substantial medical, psychological, and social impact. Transgender people face disparities in all aspects of their lives—education, employment, and health care, to name just a few. Access to bathrooms is an issue that has received fair attention. Violence against transgenders is a worrisome trend.

When people identify themselves in terms of a gender that is opposite the one assigned at birth, what role does the medical community play in the overarching scheme of things?

CHAPTER 13

IN BETWEEN AND IN PAIN

I magine that a loved one dies suddenly. You feel intense grief. Now imagine that this loved one was young and healthy. Your sorrow is crushing. Imagine that the person was intentionally killed because of his or her lifestyle—a lifestyle that was not hurting anyone. Your anguish becomes unbearable. And every time you hear or read about another victim who was murdered for the same reason as your loved one, you mourn in anguish once again. Until there comes a time when anger takes over and outrages at our inability as a society to halt the injustice that festers deeply within you. It can be very destructive.

More than seventeen hundred transgender people have been violently killed in the last seven years across the world. These are only the reported cases—underestimation by all means. More than the number, the brutality of the murders is gruesome and disturbing. Extreme aggression, mutilation, and torture are evident, and the reason behind the attacks most of the time has to do with the gender status of the victim. Even more worrisome are the increasing attacks on young people. After Brazil and Mexico, the United States has the highest reported rate of transgender homicide. War crimes against transgenders are endemic and often result in mass violence. The hostility and persecution that transgenders face is alarming. Consider these horrifying numbers: 41 percent attempt suicide, 50 percent face sexual assault, 66 percent face physical violence, and 66 percent face workplace discrimination. They have the highest HIV risk as a group, and 70 percent hide their transgender status to avoid discrimination. The most vulnerable of them are people of color and women.

My earliest memory of transgenders is as a child visiting New Delhi. While walking down a busy street with my family, I suddenly heard loud voices and turned around to see a group of garishly dressed women laden with cheap jewelry clapping their hands and shouting. Even at that age, I could recognize that something was different about these women. I was told that these are "eunuchs" or "*hijras*" who were a nuisance to our society—they would magically appear in hordes at social functions like weddings, childbirths, funerals, and store openings to demand money and gold and would create a commotion if the hosts did not oblige. People in Delhi were intensely anxious about them whenever they had an auspicious celebration. Later I would realize that this sort of extortion was their only means of sustenance; they had no other source of income.

As I grew older, I saw them on television and in movies and realized that they were "men dressed as women." In English, and later on as I found out in medicine too, they were sometimes termed "hermaphrodites"—people with ambiguous genitalia and sexual identity, not quite the same as transgender, who may have normal genitalia. In Indian movies, they either portrayed irrelevant negative characters or were the subjects of jokes in clownish comedy. Overall, there was always a negative connotation until a few years ago when I saw an Indian reality show with a prominent transgender woman, Laxmi Narayan Tripathi. Her grave demeanor, aesthetic eloquence, scholarly work, and extensive advocacy on national and international platforms took me by surprise. She was held in high esteem and regarded as a legend in her community. She spoke extensively about her struggles and the role of her conservative family in supporting her to speak up. She brought her father on the show. He had accepted her without the expected ostracizing. She is the first transgender person to represent Asia-Pacific at the United Nations. Her fame opened the window of transgenders in India to the world. Times have changed since then. Notwithstanding the slow pace, we are witnessing a turnaround, even in an ultraconservative country like India. Another interesting example that I recently witnessed was the portrayal of gay and transgender people in mainstream advertising on television, a far-reaching medium, clearly indicating a growing acceptance in the subcontinent that has high numbers of transgenders who have conventionally existed in oblivion.

The recent revelation of sixty-five-year old Olympic champion Bruce Jenner, now Caitlyn Jenner, that she was a male-to-female transgender person has brought to the forefront of American society an often-sidelined group of people who have historically struggled with social acceptance, psychological problems, economic difficulties, and inadequate access to health care. The shaming that I have personally encountered as an advocate is trivial in comparison, though being called shallow, insincere, and odd, and accusations of glamorizing what many consider "crazy acts by crazy people" is not fun. The global lack of awareness and misinformation regarding transgender people is disheartening. Until recently, the trans world has been clandestinely discussed in a salacious manner, made fun of, ridiculed, and dismissed as a fad or freak with no biological or psychological foundation whatsoever. Even the medical community has taken its time to accept that it is a "real thing" that exists, that it is a biological phenomenon. Doctors have been known to bluntly tell patients that they don't know how to provide care to a transgender person, as if they were a whole new species.

But what does transgender really mean? I felt confused myself with so many different terms used to describe transgender people. In simple words, the gender spectrum is bookended on each side by a man and a woman, and in between is a group of people whose *self-identity* does not conform to the conventional binary dyad. They are identified under the umbrella term "transgender," which includes transsexual, transvestite, cross-dressing, gender variant, gender nonspecific, gender queer, polygender, androgyne, drag queen or king, and male or female impersonators. In the past, specific definitions described each of them, but considerable overlap exists that is confusing and perhaps unnecessary, especially since some of these terms are considered derogatory.

Having worked at one of the largest LGBT (lesbian, gay, bisexual, transgender) centers for HIV disease in the Midwest, I often encountered transgenders in my practice. I found their lives incredibly complicated in every aspect—physical, mental, emotional, social, economic, and most importantly regarding health care. My concern for their safety from physical and sexual assaults gave me a peep into their world—where they sleep, what they eat, who they hang out with, and whether they have emergency contacts. Most of them were inconsistent in their clinic visits and HIV treatment. In every visit, I would discuss the importance of adherence to their HIV medicines, knowing well that they would not follow the regimen. Initially I was somewhat disapproving of the noncompliance, but as I got to know the community better, I realized that HIV was not their biggest battle—survival was.

The fundamental concept of "self-identity" defines who transgenders are. It is different from sexuality. This is the most common mistake made by nontrans people in understanding them. Self-identity is who you think you are; sexuality is who you want to be with. The unique challenges faced by this particular cohort of the population are tough to quantify or examine, since there are barely any credible statistics available, either from the state or in the practice of evidence-based medicine. I feel compelled to write about a few sobering facts that will help us understand them better and perhaps dispel an unreasonable demonization that has led to unspeakable crimes against them.

There are almost a million transgender people in the United States—the exact number is seven hundred thousand (0.3 percent of the population), but it is clearly an underestimation. The global number is unknown. Statistics are likely to be underestimations because of underreporting resulting from the stigma attached to being transgender and the usual lack of a third gender status option in census bureau reports. In recent reports, as many as one in one hundred people may have gender nonconformity, including two to four children per two thousand in schools. Transgender-related vocabulary causes confusion and unintentional distress. Gender dysphoria and gender identity disorder are often used interchangeably without correctly understanding what each of the terms means. Clubbing all transgenders under a term recognized by psychiatrists as a mental illness has received criticism as being flawed and inaccurate. However, just like homosexuality, this perception is changing as time goes by. Homosexuality was recognized as a psychiatric illness until 1973 in the *Diagnostic and Statistical Manual of Mental Disorders* (*DSM*) when the American Psychiatric Association removed it as a diagnosis of mental disease. However, it was not until 1987 that all conditions related to it were finally removed from the *DSM*. The rationale behind this volte-face was the fact that not all homosexual people are distressed by their sexual orientation and thus are psychologically healthy.

In the recently released *DSM-5*, gender identity disorder has been replaced by gender dysphoria, a strong step in understanding and describing transgender people, since not all of them can be considered mentally ill. The American Psychiatric Association has made it clear that "gender nonconformity is not in itself a mental disorder." However, completely eliminating gender-identity disorder as a diagnosis raised concerns about obstructing access to specific medical and surgical care that transgenders need under health insurance—for example, hormonal therapy, gender-reassignment surgery, psychological counseling, and other social and legal shifts mandated for full transition to the opposite sex. Thus, the term gender dysphoria has replaced gender-identity disorder.

Both of these terms refer to a state in which someone feels uncomfortable with the gender assigned at birth and identifies strongly with the opposite gender, either a male-to-female or a female-to-male. Occasionally, there are conditions in which people may have both the female and male genitals but are assigned as a boy or girl at birth. Gender-identity disorder was a term used to describe such transpeople, inadvertently labeling them all permanently as mentally sick. In reality, some transgenders do not experience any anguish, anxiety, or suffering related to their trans state and remain psychologically healthy. Recognizing this aspect of the transpeople led to the new term, gender dysphoria, which includes only those transgenders who feel distressed as a result of the incompatibility with their identity, recognizing the psychological feelings of discontent or dissatisfaction with their assigned gender. The American Psychiatric Association describes this distress as one that results in "impairment in social, occupational, or other important areas of functioning." This doesn't necessarily make them mentally ill, and gender dysphoria has been termed as a transient state for which treatment may be appropriate at times. Gender-identity disorder is a term that is no longer used. The feelings of dysphoria usually appear in early childhood. Some continue to feel the same beyond adolescence and are called persisters, while others don't and are called desisters.

One of the most remarkable manifestations of changing times was the featuring of Laverne Cox on the *TIME* cover last year. Laverne is an African American, male-to-female transgender person who stars in the epic Netflix television series *Orange is the New Black*. She was also voted as one of the top five most-influential leaders of the year. In an interesting aside, her twin brother, Lamar, also stars in the same series, playing her character as a man before her transition to a woman. When I first started watching the show, I was impressed at the character representation by Cox without knowing that she was a transgender in real life. It's a remarkable story of success—she identified as a girl when she was very young and always wanted to be famous as an actor without understanding what a high bar she was setting for herself with being black *and* transgender. That she had a tremendous support system is a notable feat in itself, considering the stigma and shame that families often experience in such situations. Chaz Bono, son of legendary singer Cher, is a familiar female-to-male-transgender activist whose strained relationship with his mother in the early part of his transition is well known. Thomas Beatie is widely known for having transitioned from a woman into a man and then proceeding to have two normal pregnancies since his uterus was preserved. Showbiz and pop culture are replete with many creative and talented transgender artists who are not just accepted in *visual* roles historically intended for the opposite gender but have also proved to be relentless in their advocacy for equity and social justice. From competing in modeling and beauty contests to playing central roles on daytime television, transpeople have proved that they can lead highly productive lives that can inspire and transform the lives of other transpeople.

One of the many impressive transgender personalities that I have read about is Dr. Marci Bowers, a world-renowned gynecologist in California, who is considered the guru of gender-reassignment surgery (GRS), having performed more than a thousand surgeries in the last decade. She is a male-to-female-transgender person and holds the record for being the first transwoman ever to perform transgender surgery. Gender-reassignment surgery involves reconstruction of the external genitalia from one gender to another. In a male-to-female GRS, the penis and testes are removed and scrotal flaps restructured to resemble a vagina and labia. The prostate is preserved and estrogen therapy is initiated to encourage feminization like breast growth, voice change, and so on. Getting breast augmentation and other head-and-neck surgeries, such as shaving of the Adam's apple and recreating feminine facial features, is a personal choice. In a female-to-male GRS, the clitoris is enlarged to resemble a penis, either hormonally using testosterone or with grafts from other parts of the body and a prosthesis in a reconstructive procedure called phalloplasty. The uterus and ovaries are removed unless the person wants to preserve them, as in the case of Thomas Beatie. Male hormones deepen the voice and boost hirsutism, or growth of body hair. Breast-reduction surgery is done to add to the masculinity.

There are no reliable sources to report exactly how many GRS procedures are done every year in the United States, partly because of the surreptitious nature of the condition. There are easily several hundred that are reported. It is an expensive surgery, with the female-to-male procedure costing more than twice the male-to-female one, and affordability is obviously a big issue, with or without health insurance. Prognostically, the former is less successful because of the challenges associated with enlarging a small clitoris to a much larger and functional penis. Dr. Bowers is a strong supporter of GRS being done at a young age when the patients can still receive support from their family system. She is highly sought after globally for teaching complex GRS techniques in different parts of the world. Dr. Bowers is also well known for her pioneering work in the rehabilitation of women who suffered genital mutilation for whom she does reversal surgery free of cost. What better example could there be of a vibrant, dynamic transgender innovator who has made a difference in the lives of others with her prolific creativity in health care?

In politics, Europe has seen prominent transgender persons, for example, in Italy and Poland. Vladimir Luxuria is an Italian male-to-female-transgender person who is the first transperson to become a member of the European Parliament. She was born a man and lives as a woman, though she has not had GRS as she does not want to be addressed as either a man or a woman. There is a subgroup of transpeople who identify neither as man nor as woman. *Nonspecific*-gender status does not get recognition in most countries of the world including the United States and thus they have negligible legal rights. Asian countries have taken a lead in this matter, which is quite fascinating to ponder. Only seven countries in the world recognize an "other" gender legally, including Nepal, India, Pakistan, Bangladesh, Germany, New Zealand, and Australia. In fact, Nepal was the first country in the world to introduce an "other" gender status in census records for nonbinary citizens. Germany now allows parents to choose an undetermined gender when a child is born, if there is ambiguity about gender, so that the child can have an option to choose when he or she grows up. Nonbinary status in these countries still does not provide the same rights to transgender people in all walks of life, and much progress is hoped for in the future. Western countries like United States are far behind in this matter in spite of the sometimes-intense public spotlight on the rising prominence of transgender figures.

Transgenders face the same health problems and concerns as the general population. In addition, they are challenged by disparities unique to them that stem from social stigma, resulting in marginalization. The situation becomes more perilous when they belong to multiple minority groups based on race, ethnicity, religion, and nationality. Because of distinctive lifestyle and psychosocial factors, they have a higher prevalence of chronic disorders like obesity and mental illness as well as sexually transmitted diseases, including HIV. They tend to become disabled at an earlier age for many reasons, especially because they have poor access to primary care and seek little, if any, preventive medical care like screening for cancer with colonoscopy and mammography. The awkwardness of going to visit a doctor in a regular office among nontransgenders is a deterrent in seeking help because of the low level of comfort and prohibitive fees in the absence of health insurance. Health-care providers not adequately trained in addressing unique health issues may inadvertently provide insufficient treatment, advice, or counseling.

Health-insurance coverage is a gray zone that is poorly defined—transgender persons may be eligible for public aid based on their annual income, which may not pay for hormonal treatment, GRS, or psychological counseling. There has been a slow change in the last few years, said Dr. Bowers on the *Dr. Drew Show* recently. Twelve years ago, no insurance companies covered surgeries for transgender transition. Now nine US states are looking at insurance coverage for some, but not all, of the treatments and surgeries.

Two-thirds of working transgender people face serious discrimination at work. Any remote physical attribute that may give away their gender status becomes a reason not to hire, say most transgender persons. Employment opportunities are scarce; consequently, employment-based insurance is sporadic at best and often driven by geographical variables. For example, the liberal culture of California provides a more comfortable environment for transgenders, and with it comes equity in jobs and other opportunities. The conservative Midwest may be more challenging. Hopefully, the new Supreme Court ruling lifting the ban on same-sex marriage will result in broader coverage in domestic partnerships, but the ambiguity in legal gender-status recognition causes uncertainty and an absence of uniformity in partner benefits. Lack of health literacy leads to poor health-care utilization. Hospital visits are not easily accessible because of strict rules and regulations. These factors drive transgenders to ignore their health until they are very sick or to find illicit medical care that is inappropriate, dangerous, and even life threatening, like street estrogen for feminization. According to the American College of Physicians (ACP), "These laws and policies, along with others that reinforce marginalization, discrimination, social stigma, or rejection of LGBT persons by their families or communities or that simply keep LGBT persons from accessing health care, have been associated with increased rates of anxiety, suicide, and substance or alcohol abuse."

The transgender community is at the highest risk for HIV disease in the country, and a worrisome majority is unaware of their status. According to the Centers for Disease Control (CDC), newly diagnosed HIV-positive tests are seen in transgender persons in higher numbers than nontransgender persons. African American transgender persons had four times the incidence of white transgender persons, and Hispanic transgender persons had three times the incidence of white transgender persons. Globally, HIV prevalence in transgender women is fifty times higher than any other adult group—a horrifying statistic. Unfortunately, many of them are homeless, unemployed, and have a history of incarceration, sexual abuse, and substance abuse. This is in keeping with my LGBT experience in Chicago—transgender folks are compelled to become sex workers as a means of living because of discrimination in education and employment, and they are often abused in many ways. Poor public-health policies, social prejudices, insensitive health-care providers, inadequate training in cultural competency, and a lack of statistical data increase the complexity of transgender persons with HIV disease. Access to long-term specialty care is fragmented that may translate into delays in diagnosis and treatment.

One of the unique medical problems that male-to-female transgender persons face involves drug interactions if they have other chronic disorders like HIV, hypertension, and diabetes—for example, several anti-HIV medicines interact with estrogen that may be part of their feminizing hormonal treatment. Estrogen increases the risk for blood clots and stroke. I remember reading about a well-known transgender person in Chicago who died of a stroke that was believed to have been caused by high levels of estrogen. She was HIV positive and was on an anti-HIV combination regimen. Since a few of these drugs increase metabolism of estrogen by the liver, the prescribed dose of estrogen had to be increased. Later she stopped taking her HIV medicines for unknown reasons but continued to take the higher dose of estrogen instead of reducing it which could have been the reason for the stroke. Many transwomen have access to street estrogen only because of a lack of health insurance which is more dangerous because of impurities.

Such unfortunate incidents are not uncommon and indicate a health-care disparity within the community.

"Transphobia" is widespread all over the world. Bullying and violence in their many forms—verbal, physical, mental, sexual—are social stressors that most transgender persons have to face early on in their lives. The tenuous social dynamics make transgender persons easy victims of intimate-partner violence. Bathroom privileges are a common problem. Public beatings of transgender persons who use women's bathrooms has happened. A list of transgender persons killed unlawfully in the last three decades can be found at https://en.wikipedia.org/wiki/List_of_unlawfully_killed_transgender_people. "Fetishizing" is another accusation that they face on a regular basis—objectifying yourself with makeup and dresses to attract negative attention. They are not welcome to enroll in the army and seek GRS-related treatment. Transgender inmates in correctional health facilities face health-care disparities too. They are universally denied GRS and have widely variable access to other treatments, including hormonal therapy. Shiloh Heavenly Quine became the first inmate to receive GRS in the United Sates recently. Though outrage at the $100,000 treatment provided to a murderer erupted across the country, her struggle with gender identity represents what this community consistently suffers from. From all accounts, she was so severely depressed about her gender that she tried to commit suicide several times in the prison.

The American College of Physicians (ACP) has strongly advocated that LGBT-related health issues be incorporated into the medical-school curriculum, and their community in general should be encouraged to actively participate and integrate with the medical community. Medical students are ill prepared to care for certain aspects of LGBT health, and concerns regarding transgender care are evident in surveys across medical schools. Cultural competency is the need of the hour for all levels of health-care providers to successfully integrate the health care of gender-nonconforming individuals. For example, those who transition from one gender to another pose a confusing question about cancer screening—should we screen for breast cancer with mammography in a female-to-male transgender who still has breasts? What about those who underwent a bilateral mastectomy? Breast care is associated with considerable risks because of other procedures that transgender persons undergo, such as implants, binding, injections, and so on. The same can be said for Pap smears for screening for cervical cancer. Literature is not yet replete with evidence one way or another, so patients may fall through the cracks and not get adequate care. Tailoring the teaching of medical students to understand and care for gender-variant patients from the get-go will be critical in mitigating the disparity of this vulnerable community. One of the limitations of conducting research on a gender-nonconforming population is that because of the stigma that comes with disclosing participants' identities, investigators may be confronted with the lack of a large sample to study. It has been reported that transgender people often feel more comfortable in discussing health needs and resources anonymously on social media like twitter rather than overtly in clinics and hospitals, which are the traditional sources of data for research. Utilizing social media for data collection through surveys has been postulated as an innovative way to conduct useful research. More transgender professionals in the medical field would certainly help to bridge the chasm of communication and promote inclusivity.

One of the key criticisms that LGBT supporters face is the difference in LGB and transgender patronage—though they are lumped together under the umbrella term, they are not the same and have disparate needs. LGBT advocacy groups, including physicians, have often accused the World Health Organization (WHO)

and other global peer institutions of neglecting the health disparities faced by transgender folks across the world while reinforcing
gay rights, thus not fulfilling their core responsibility of ensuring
equal access to health services by all groups of people without discrimination. However, the director general of WHO, Margaret
Chan, indicated a paradigm shift in the approach of the organization toward transgender health when she spoke at the 2015
executive-board session. She said that "there is growing evidence
that well-functioning and inclusive health systems contribute to social cohesion, equity, and stability." It is anticipated that WHO will
lead from the front when it comes to establishing fair parameters
for the human rights of transgender persons, including appropriate health care and access to affordable high-quality care.

History has taught us that at regular intervals in time, human beings have emerged in uprisings to fight for and protect an
underprivileged minority of society—like women, blacks, homo-
sexuals, and so on—against the tyranny of the dominant social
order. These battles have been variously called civil war, revolution, mutiny, riot, insurgence, and so on, though the central theme
has always been the same. This time, it is the turn of transgender
people. They have been in existence since time immemorial but
have lived in a distorted world of prejudice and inequity. The Dalai
Lama once said to be kind whenever possible. It's always possible.
We, as a society, have the responsibility to care for one another and
be accepting of who we are as individuals and as people. Honestly,
it doesn't take much to stand up for those who are constantly bul-
lied, beaten up, murdered, or driven to suicide. Criminal-law protection for transgender people for the considerable perpetration
of violence against them has to be a prime agenda of global political, legal, advocacy, and diplomatic agencies. An encouraging sign
of progress was the new birth certificate of fifty-five-year-old Sara
Kelly Keenan. It describes her gender as "Intersex" rather than

male or female. She was born with female external genitalia, male genes, and a mix of male and female internal reproductive organs.

Franklin Roosevelt, a remarkable statesman and past president of United States, once said, "In these days of difficulty, we Americans everywhere must and shall choose the path of social justice, the path of faith, the path of hope, and the path of love toward our fellow man." Decades later, these words remain strangely apt for transgender health in America and worldwide. Though alternate sexual orientation has become widely accepted in our society, gender identity remains poorly acknowledged. Health insurance for transgender people's unique needs will be a complex topic for a long time, just like it has been for everyone else in the United States—a crisis of monstrous proportions.

CHAPTER 14

THE LOCH NESS MONSTER

Emily was a forty-six-year-old woman whom I met only once in my clinic at a public hospital. She was a tall, statuesque Caucasian woman who was soft-spoken and incredibly articulate, an unusual combination at the institution where I worked and mostly took care of the multiethnic vulnerable population. For the next two years, Emily called me on my phone almost on a weekly basis, each time with a different clinical question left on my voice mail or with my staff. Every conversation was a series of quirky queries, sometimes bordering on the bizarre that I politely tried to answer to the best of my abilities. When I first met her, she was uninsured. But within a couple of months, she was able to get enrolled in Medicaid under the Affordable Care Act (ACA), which was implemented a year and a half ahead of the expected schedule in my hospital. In fact, she was one of the first enrollees in the state.

Like a switch being turned on, something seemed to click in her mind—she now had health insurance, something she had not had for a very long time. In fact, I am not sure if she ever had health insurance in her life. With coverage came expectations. When could she get a colonoscopy? Though she was not yet fifty (when the usual screening for colon cancer begins), she wanted to get an early start and not wait for another four years. When could she consult an orthopedic specialist for arthritis of her hip? The symptoms were mild, and I could take care of it as her primary-care physician, but she thought she may choose a hip replacement now instead of waiting till it gets really bad. How soon can she get an MRI of the brain? She didn't really have any symptoms; she just wanted to ensure there were no early findings of dementia that she had read about. Now that she had health insurance, she wanted to be tested for "poisons" in her blood like arsenic and other metals. Could I refer her to our lab for those tests? If the lab didn't do these tests, then could I put in an order for the phlebotomist in the lab to draw her blood and give her the vials so that she could mail them to another lab in Ohio that performs these tests? When I said no, we cannot do that, she said, "Why not? After all, it's my blood. I should be able to do whatever I want to do with it. And now I have insurance that should pay for it."

And so on, and so forth—the requests got more peculiar as time passed. She missed every clinic appointment that she scheduled. On the phone, I had extensive discussions with her about screening guidelines and appropriateness of tests based on clinical symptoms and signs on physical examination. Most of my advice was ignored and she openly expressed her disagreement with the standard indications for tests that she requested. She demanded that one way or another she should be able to get the care that she wanted. I tried to explain to her the limitations of Medicaid under ACA that it was still a new process and we were trying to figure out how it works, the referrals for preventive care and screenings, specialists, complex surgeries, and so on—basically all the care that was not provided at our institution or had a long waiting list. Some private practices, or most of them, refuse to accept patients with Medicaid, especially specialists and superspecialists. She couldn't quite understand how that was possible. How can they do that? After all, "it's the president's insurance. No one should be allowed to refuse Obamacare."

Then there was Mr. Johnson, a Vietnam War veteran who had not been to a doctor for almost a decade. He scheduled an appointment with me in my suburban practice for shortness of breath and leg swelling. Within a few minutes, I knew he was very sick and needed to be hospitalized immediately. It could be heart failure, blood clots in his legs and lungs, coronary artery disease, or a few other life-threatening conditions. However, he adamantly refused a hospital admission. Even though he was enrolled in Medicare, he would have to pay a coinsurance. This was the main reason why he had abstained from seeking care with a primary-care physician or specialist. Twenty percent of the bill (his share) was not affordable for him. He had waited to get really sick to avoid medical bills that would have fleeced him of the small social-security check that he got monthly. I discussed the chain of Veteran's Affairs (VA) hospitals that would have probably cost him nothing or at least not as much. All things considered, the United States boasts of "the most comprehensive assistance for veterans in the world." He had a poor understanding of the VA system and thought it would cost him a lot too. And anyway, there were no VA hospitals within a radius of fifty miles of his home, and he could not afford to commute frequently to the nearest one, which was sixty miles away. He lived alone and had no family or friends who could help him. Simply put, he just could not afford to get sick.

Maria Guadalupe was thirty-seven years old and an undocumented immigrant from Mexico. She had moved to the United States five years ago with her two children, a boy and a girl, both teenagers now. She was unmarried and lived with her boyfriend, also Mexican. Unfortunately, she was diagnosed with metastatic anal cancer approximately a year ago that had made her so sick that she spent a majority of the time admitted in the hospital for long stretches interspersed with brief home discharges, a vicious cycle that drained her tiny family of all their resources. She had fluid-filled lungs that made her breathing shallow and painful. She had numerous tubes from her body, including a urinary catheter, anal tubes, multiple intravenous sites, and a port for chemotherapy. Her last hospital admission was close to two months in duration during which she got better enough several times to go home but refused discharge, as there was no one to take care of her other than her children (her boyfriend was at work for long hours). Social workers reviewed her housing status and confirmed the same—she would come right back to the emergency room with the slightest deterioration in her already precarious disposition. Palliative services tried to arrange a skilled-nursing-facility transfer for her, but she was ineligible for it, not because she had no insurance but because she was undocumented. Home-hospice care had the same issue. So she continued to be at the hospital until she passed away. Seeing her immense suffering daily, including intractable pain, the medical team felt a sense of relief for her sake, even though the sadness of the circumstances was not lost on any of us. We worried about her children. But they both seemed surprisingly well adjusted and were on good terms with her boyfriend, who would become their primary guardian. Her entire care had cost the hospital system close to a million dollars that would remain unreimbursed.

Sandra was fifty-two years old and had mild diabetes and hypothyroidism, both of which were well controlled. She was single and employed, had her own home and no children. Her employer provided her with good private-health insurance that had a set copay per office visit, a $2,000 deductible per year, and 20 percent coinsurance for hospital, lab, radiology, surgery, and other bills—a pretty good deal at a cursory glance. Six months after I first met her in my suburban private practice, she was diagnosed with an aggressive maxillary sinus cancer that required a complicated facial surgery, intense radiation treatment, as well as chemotherapy. Over the next few months, I watched in utter dismay a beautiful woman's face turn into a swollen, horrific, scar-ridden open wound with an unbearable stench of rotting tissue. Soon, she was unable to swallow and had a gastric tube placed for nutrition through which she did bolus feeding three times a day. She had poor to negligible social support and had to stop driving, as the changing anatomical configuration below one eye pushed at her orbital tissues to affect her vision. But the worst part of this story was the toll it took on her mental and emotional health. As if the cancer wasn't enough to cause anxiety, she had other problems to worry about—losing her job, losing her health insurance, being unable to pay her medical bills on time and going bankrupt. She could lose her house and fretted about her personal expenses that included a mortgage. Eventually she was able to get a home-equity loan that could pay for her needs briefly. She became dependent on neighbors and friends to drive her to her many doctors' visits or paid for an expensive cab ride. Social workers anticipated that at some point she could possibly qualify for Medicaid or disability, but not anytime soon.

These real cases are examples of how complex and disastrous the byzantine American health-care system currently is. The grim reality of each of these patients reflects the calamitous nature of health-insurance coverage. Countless "insured" Americans like Sandra are ill informed about what their medical bills are likely to be, either for preventive services or after a sickness or surgery. To make matters worse, it is nearly impossible to get that information from the insurance company, the doctors' offices, or the hospitals. I recently read about a highly placed pregnant lawyer who tried to find out how much it would cost her to have her baby. After innumerable phone calls and hours on the phone, she was still at square one with no clue. The situation is as precarious for the insured as it is for the underinsured and uninsured—medical bills can lead to bankruptcy, and in fact, it is the leading cause of bankruptcy nationwide. Health insurance is like a colossal jungle teeming with people, none of whom know the way out of the jungle—you can stop as many of them as you like to ask for directions, and the standard answer will be "I don't know." As an active physician in the United States since 1998, I am embarrassed to say that I know or understand health insurance inadequately myself, and I daresay that not more than a handful of medical personnel comprehend it in its entirety. Most of my colleagues will agree with me.

Why is it so? Does it have to be so complex? Who established this intricate and convoluted system that has spun out of control into a bewildering maze of interlocking, labyrinthine, and frequently obscure networks that trap patients, physicians, employers, administrators, and healthcare executives alike? Personally, I have experienced its confusing existence in all these roles during different periods in my life. It was equally incomprehensible every single time.

Emily represents the intrinsic mind-set that once we have insurance coverage we achieve some sort of health-care nirvana. We somehow become liberated from the shackles of our insecurities about health and illness. Of course, our access to care improves radically. We can now choose to consult a doctor, any doctor; get tests, any tests; perform X-rays, any X-rays; buy medicines, any medicines; and so on. This falsehood has been generated since time immemorial and we, as customers, fall into that trap repeatedly. No, we cannot consult any doctor that we want, or get any test that suits our fancy, or buy any medication that we deem appropriate. In most ways, this is a good thing—we must follow guidelines for standardization, uniform care delivery, appropriateness of services, and to prevent misuse. Otherwise, everyone would want to check levels of metals in their blood and request an MRI for minor symptoms! But it also limits and complicates our options as patients—the in-network confusion, capitation conundrum, enigmatic service fees, mystery-riddled explanations of benefits, and surprise charges, to name a few. We need a simple system that explains benefits and costs clearly and allows patients to compare services online, just like we do for other things, like buying a car or a house and shopping online. We also need to dispel the belief that having insurance coverage is like having manna from heaven—neither was it before the ACA nor will it be after. There are no entitlements promised and none will be delivered.

As far as veterans are concerned, they form a distinctive section of our society with unique health-care needs that we must address unambiguously. Vietnam warriors form the largest veteran group in the United States and have limitations just like Mr. Johnson. Commuting to a VA hospital is a major problem. Providing them with discounted transportation either as a specific service or as part of their health-care coverage is necessary to ensure access to care. Under the ACA, enrollees are qualified to get transportation to and from their health-care-related visits, a critical benefit that I personally found very useful for many of my patients. Vets should be provided with this benefit too. Home health-physician visits are another solution to the problem of access for veterans. A network of providers trained in military culture and exposures during war could be engaged to provide affordable, high-quality care to our veterans in need. Reimbursement of these providers should be such that it attracts skilled physicians to consider it as a viable career option that includes administrative and commuting costs.

The ACA has brought about many positive changes since its implementation. Under its scope, thirty million people will eventually be able to get health-insurance coverage with Medicaid expansion. The "preexisting medical condition" clause used by private companies to deny coverage has been removed. Community rating ensures that insurance companies do not charge higher premiums based on health status or impose lifetime caps on coverage. Tax credits for those meeting the criteria for income is a critical provision. Medicare coverage has been improved to decrease the cost of prescription medications and remove copayments for preventive care. Opposition to the ACA among Americans is based largely on the directive that health insurance is mandatory for everyone—the individual mandate. I am somewhat puzzled by this since Medicare, which is mandatory for those above age sixty-five, has huge support among Americans. Researchers have blamed aggressive Republican-backed television advertising against the ACA as the principal reason behind it. Overall though, it has mostly had a positive impact, though it remains peppered with snags and hitches.

After fifty years since the inception of Medicare and Medicaid, there are fifty-five million enrollees in Medicare and seventy million in Medicaid. Whether the ACA will result in long-term, meaningful reform is still to be seen. Certainly, broadening the coverage to include millions of patients is an inherently well-intentioned step. I recently interviewed Dr. Alice Chen, the executive director of Doctors for America. The organization was founded by Dr. Vivek Murthy, the US surgeon general who spearheaded the implementation of the ACA with President Barack Obama. Several things struck me as noteworthy in my conversation with Dr. Chen, one of which was that "nobody wins when people are sick." This powerful statement is so simple, yet so profoundly expressive. The bottom line is that the sicker we are, the higher the cost of care.

Appropriate care when *needed* rather than when we are the sickest is vital and fundamental to improve overall health and reduce cost.

Recently, the state of California budgeted millions of dollars to cover children of undocumented immigrants under Medi-Cal, the Medicaid version of the state under the ACA. Soon undocumented adults will also be able to come under its purview if they meet certain income criteria. This has caused a certain degree of anxiety and heartburn among some American citizens. How and why should we have to spend tax dollars for undocumented immigrants? The truth is that one way or another we will have to pay for their medical care when they are sick—they live in the United States and work here. They pay taxes on consumer products and their salaries, often with fake social-security numbers that means their contribution to Medicare is lost money for them. They provide services that perhaps legal citizens may not want to. If they do not have health insurance, they will not be able to get care when needed but will wait until they are too sick and need emergency care, which will decidedly be more expensive. "Episodic acute care" is the term that describes this type of medical care, and it has been proven without a doubt that it results in poor outcomes and is a strain on already stretched resources. If Maria Guadalupe had Medicaid, we would have been able to provide her with many services like home health care, nursing-home care, and hospice care. Instead of lingering in the hospital with terminal cancer, she would have been able to be home or in a nursing home, and the cost of care would have been a fraction of what it turned out to be—a win-win situation. As Dr. Chen pointed out, how can we as a society decide that we will pay for health care for a section of the community and not for those who were born in another country? This is not what America is all about. Immigrants are the core of the American identity, and until we have legislation that controls illegal immigration, we are ethically and morally bound as health-care providers to care for those already residing in the United States, regardless of any political inclination. And yes—it will be much more cost-effective for us to do that.

Long-term care remains a setting where we have seen marginal reform. Patients either pay out of pocket or are enrolled in Medicaid when their money runs out. Caring for the aging baby boomers is a key issue that requires keen coordination of services because of increasing demand as life expectancy increases. According to the Centers for Disease Control, one in five adults has a disability in the United States. Medicare reform is the need of the hour, but a distant reality. It is fraught with problems that need urgently to be fixed. Though Medicare enrollees represent less than 12 percent of the population in the United States, they expend 40 percent of the medications, and part D for medications is neither the most efficient nor adequate approach to providing benefits. Part B for outpatient care carries a copay that is often unaffordable for enrollees, even in small dollar amounts. Medicare has been pronounced on life support for more than a decade. Soon it will be time to either pull the plug or try another remedy.

Emily remained unseen at my clinic and mysteriously was able to get herself tested for "metal poisons." Of course, I was concerned about her mental health and discussed options subtly with her, but there was no way to refer her to a psychiatrist without seriously offending her and losing her entirely. The irony of the situation was that under the ACA she would have access to mental-health services more easily than before. Mr. Johnson passed away from complications of his long-standing, underlying conditions soon after I met him. If only he had sought care five years earlier, he would still be alive. Sandra struggled bravely with her cancer and was declared cancer-free though her facial anatomy was permanently distorted. She lost her job and ran out of her savings. The last time

I saw her, she was working with the social worker to apply for disability. Life was never going to be the same for her again.

There are so many problems and few solutions. In my opinion, the most critical issue remains *access* to affordable, high-quality, medical care for all-population groups. Innovation in health care is the need of the day. How can we improve access to care in a way that improves health outcomes without disrupting the patient-physician relationship but is also in sync with the technological revolution that is happening across the globe? Perhaps *telemedicine* is one of the answers.

CHAPTER 15
SO FAR, YET SO CLOSE

"Hello?"

"Hi! May I speak to Laura Kepple, please? This is Dr. Pandey."

"Hi, Dr. Pandey. How are you?"

"Good morning! I am well, thank you. You requested an online consultation with me. What can I do for you today?"

"Dr. Pandey, I had a tick bite on my right arm a week ago and removed the tick myself. There is a rash around it, and I have uploaded a picture for you to review. I am worried about Lyme disease since I was in Connecticut. I can feel a lump in my right armpit that is a little tender to touch. What should I do? I am at work and cannot take a day off to go to the doctor right away."

Laura is one of hundreds of thousands of Americans who are choosing to get medical care via telemedicine—using technology to get remote delivery of health-care services. She had little time to take off from work to go to the doctor's office, and she was mostly interested in getting information about what to do next. She read about Lyme disease on the Internet and had a fair understanding of the basic steps to take after a tick bite to rule out Lyme disease. All she wanted was information from a health-care provider who could answer some of her questions. Once she had all the information, she would be able to make an informed decision about taking time off to schedule an appointment with her primary-care physician who may want to do blood tests or prescribe medication.

Personally, I had an inherent problem with providing medical services virtually—how can your assessment be complete without a physical examination? However, as I better understood the entire scope of telemedicine, I changed my mind and have been in the process of comprehending the assortment of services that can be provided as well as the upside of merging technology with medicine. Innovative service-delivery systems and online-business models use telephones, videos, webcams, and state-of-the-art medical equipment for virtual physical examinations including otoscope, fundoscope, stethoscope, and so on to provide remote health care to patients in different settings, including intensive care, urgent care, chronic care, disease monitoring, second opinions, and so on.

In a bittersweet way, the traditional practice of medicine is fading away into oblivion as solo and small practices struggle with the burden of integrating health information technology at significant costs as well as recent regulatory restrictions that have been overwhelming in general for the medical community. This has affected the doctor-patient relationship, and patients can no longer have the security of being able to reach their family doctors whenever needed. On the other hand, within a matter of minutes, they could potentially have a health-care provider on the telephone or video who is in all likelihood living in another state or city but could assist them by answering questions, making decisions, and even prescribing some medications electronically.

The American Telemedicine Association (ATA) defines telemedicine (sometimes called telehealth) as "the remote delivery of health-care services using telecommunications technology: Internet, wireless services, satellite, and telephone media." Telemedicine services have been available for over forty years in the United States. In its current dimension, it encompasses several aspects of medical care:

- Delivering clinical services from a health-care provider to a patient in a different location via telephone, video, or webcam for urgent care
- E-mailing communication between doctor and patient for nonurgent health-related issues
- Maintaining patient-driven, electronic health records to share with providers as needed using smartphone apps to track your health
- Managing chronic disease by using remote monitoring equipment
- Getting second opinions
- Using specialists like radiologists to read imaging tests remotely

These are only a few examples of telemedicine, the scope of which is far wider. Interest in telemedicine has been revived in the last few years because of many reasons. According to the ATA, more than fifteen million American will receive remote care consultations in 2015, including twelve thousand stroke patients and five hundred thousand ICU patients. Cost of care, access to care, and insurance coverage are a few problems that have been addressed by telemedicine. A burgeoning baby-boomer population, with a longer life expectancy than ever before and multiple chronic disorders, in need of continuous care with high medical costs, has spurred ways to take care of them without compromising either the quality of care or the cost. On the other hand, the millennial generation is much less inclined to go to see a doctor, growing up as they are immersed in the Internet and social media. Engaging them to care for their health can be difficult, and using social media, text messaging, video, and telephone in a structured telemedicine program has been a strategic focus of Kaiser Permanente in California.

According to the *Journal of the American Medical Association*, studies have reported that 25 percent to 70 percent of office visits to see the doctor may not need a face-to-face appointment, and communication over the telephone, e-mail, or video may be adequate to resolve issues. This could lead to overall reduction in the cost of health care as well as other benefits like saving time for patients, freeing up doctors to see more patients who really need help, and decluttering the office front desk. However, the medical community has been sharply divided at times regarding the appropriateness of these virtual services, not just with the utility and suitability of care given but also reimbursement for providers for time spent in remote care that has historically not been compensated by insurance companies or patients. Regulatory policy, privacy and confidentiality issues, interstate licensing, electronic medical records, physician-to-physician communication, interoperability of electronic operating systems, and other factors have further complicated matters. Moreover, evidence in literature is also conflicting—some studies show no difference, some show reduction in costs and fewer office visits, while others show an increase in office visits because of virtual communication between doctors and patients via text or e-mail. Physicians need to be licensed in the state that they provide care. Many telemedicine doctors are thus licensed in multiple states.

With a net worth of more than $12 billion, Dr. Patrick Soon Shiong, a pioneer in telemedicine, was named by *Forbes* magazine as the world's richest doctor. In his stellar career as a highly esteemed surgeon, researcher, entrepreneur, innovator, and philanthropist, he has been an ardent exponent of the use of technology in health care. He developed highly sophisticated equipment for remote use by patients, doctors, pharmacists, and researchers. In his keynote speech at the Twentieth Annual American Telemedicine Association Trade Show in Los Angeles in May 2015 (that I personally attended), he stressed the phenomenal rise of telemedicine and use of technology in medical services. He talked about how during his "grant days," he received a grant from NASA and was part of the space-shuttle program in which the health of the astronauts in space was monitored wirelessly. He further said that he believed that it was entirely possible to do the same for everybody with the latest technological advances, and that coordination of care with the current complexities present in health care is only possible via telemedicine using current computing and technology.

Dr. Shiong addressed the extraordinary medical advances in the past five years that have made it possible for physicians to keep track of the best care available to patients. He went on to describe what he termed "predictive modeling." It is defined as the capacity to measure the human physiology and pathology at the cellular level to understand the proteins and processes that cause disease with the use of augmented intelligence. This can provide a strong clinical-decision-support system remotely or directly to health-care providers across the world to best coordinate their care. This would be the ultimate benefit of telemedicine for medical practices and patients in the not-so-distant future.

When I was enrolled in the master of public health program in medical informatics from 2006 to 2008, I read repeatedly that soon doctors, including residents and medical students, will be seen carrying handheld devices to work to coordinate care through portable computation. I found it too far-fetched at that time and could not envision such a scenario. Within a few years, however, that observation was proven right, and now we rarely see any physician without a tablet device, delivering care on the go. Dr. Shiong's predictive modeling theory may just be a possibility in the near future, when providers will have at their fingertips the latest evidence-based care guidelines with real-time coordination with multiple specialists who could drive their care to impressive levels at a fraction of the cost and time that it takes today.

Urgent Care

The advent and ubiquitous presence of handheld mobile devices like smartphones and tablets in current times have facilitated the interest in telemedicine not only in the medical community but also among software and hardware vendors, corporate professionals, the networking world, business owners, hospitals and health systems, and health-insurance companies. Patients like Laura are now able to talk to a health-care provider on smartphones and tablet devices via wireless Internet connection as and when the need arises.

This is a revolutionary concept that has improved access to care tremendously. In the past, smoking-cessation quit lines have been considered one of the few virtual services that are clinically effective and reimbursed by health-insurance companies. Telephone counseling has been proven to be a strong support system for smokers and often works as a multidisciplinary team of nurses, counselors, and social workers. The question this type of care delivery has raised is why not other services too? Acute conditions like sinusitis, the common cold, urinary-tract infections, back pain, minor injuries, skin rash, and so on can be taken care of via telemedicine. Teladoc Inc. is one of the first companies to provide remote care and is the preferred program for many health-insurance companies like Blue Shield of California. At the ATA 2015 conference, Dr. Robert Bernstein of Carena Medical Providers in Seattle, Washington, shared that cystitis and upper-respiratory infections have been proved to have better outcomes in telemedicine than with usual care in a doctor's office.

CVS MinuteClinic
MinuteClinics are walk-in clinics within CVS pharmacies, the largest pharmacy chain across United States. They provide urgent care by hiring nurse practitioners and physician assistants who are trained in managing minor family-health issues. In recent times, a few of these clinics have developed an innovative delivery system to give the patient a choice to either wait in line for the provider on site or choose a second option to be connected to a provider remotely without wasting time in the waiting rooms. Most of these clinics are in Texas and California. Dr. Tobias Barker, vice president of medical operations, spoke about their current strategic focus on the development of this telehealth program at the ATA 2015 conference in Los Angeles.

The clinics have room A (with the provider inside) or room B (with a computer monitor). The walk-in patients have the choice of waiting for room A for a provider visit or room B with a remote visit in real time. Those who choose room B get their vitals taken by a medical assistant and then are connected to a provider virtually with whom they can communicate in real time on the screen. The medical assistant remains in the room and follows directions given by the remote provider—for example, a throat swab for a rapid strep test in a patient with sore throat and fever. Otoscopes and penlights assist in the provider examining the throat or ears with the help of the medical assistant. Some facilities even have a stethoscope-like instrument that can transmit heart sounds and breath sounds to the provider. This type of program has been shown to save time and money for patients and has very high satisfaction rates.

Tele-ICU

Telemedicine services for intensive care have led the way for the rest of us. Tele-ICU has been around for many years and has been shown to reduce mortality, cost of care, and complications that are inherent in intensive-care units in hospitals. This has been most useful for remote areas where hiring intensivists is too expensive, and an open ICU is the norm—the admitting physician takes care of the patient and consults specialists as needed. These physicians are mostly family practice or internal medicine trained and may not have the necessary ICU skills. Hiring remotely placed critical-care specialists for monitoring ICU patients in underserved areas has been a trend that has curbed health-care spending to care for the increasing volume of aging patients.

Chronic Disease Care

Furthermore, evidence is accumulating that telemedicine services for chronic diseases like diabetes, hypertension, and mental disorders are also clinically effective and contain costs, especially by reducing hospital admissions. Specific evidence exists for therapeutic lifestyle changes that control and prevent diabetes like exercise, weight loss, and blood-sugar control as well as screening for diabetic retinopathy with eye examinations. Home blood-pressure telemonitoring reduces blood pressure more than usual care in which patients visit their primary-care physician two to three times a year, especially in those with target organ diseases like coronary artery disease and heart failure as well as coexisting diabetes and poor adherence to a treatment regimen. It is well accepted by patients and improves their quality of life. High technology-related costs are offset by a reduction in the cost of medical care.

Managing diabetes in a multidisciplinary approach with a physician, diabetes nurse, dietitian, and so on is also more feasible via telemedicine. Both of these conditions are highly prevalent in the United States, and poor control is common. If remote monitoring of blood pressure and blood sugar can be done without raising the cost of care and resultant improvement in clinical outcomes, then this is a win-win situation. The potential for this type of care is huge and with the right resources and leadership, telemonitoring may become the standard of care for other chronic diseases too, like emphysema, obesity, stroke, injuries, and so on.

Kristi Henderson is the chief telehealth and innovation officer at the University of Mississippi Medical Center in Jackson, Mississippi. Among other telemedicine-based platforms developed by her team, one program provides diabetes patients with an Intel tablet on which they answer questions daily regarding their blood-sugar level, medications, and so on. The data is sent to a twenty-four-hour, remote-monitoring center from where care is coordinated virtually by a team of physicians, nurses, dieticians, and so on. Mississippi currently has the second-highest prevalence of diabetes in the United States and is considered to be in a state of crisis with rising costs of care and worsening access. Governor Phil Bryant has actively supported this program in a novel effort to improve diabetes care and curtail costs. This eighteen-month program was started in the spring of 2015 and will hopefully become a prototype for future telemedicine-based programs in other states and for chronic conditions.

Second Opinions
Second opinions can be sought for cancer treatment and other conditions via telemedicine. It has been proven that 65 percent of patients who sought a second opinion about their condition changed their original treatment plan with better outcomes. Telehealth

companies like Second Opinion Expert provide access to a broad array of specialists for a fee. Patients upload their history and investigational documents into an electronic, medical-record platform and are able to connect with a specialist of their choice who reviews their records and provides a succinct second opinion. This opens the possibilities of a worldwide system of second opinions. Patients in the developing countries can get second opinions from doctors in the United States for a fraction of the cost that they would incur if they had to travel. No doubt, limitations to such care do exist, like access to a computer, Internet connection, and language barriers. Regardless, these services are likely to become very popular among patients and their families, and are highly regarded within the medical community.

Reimbursement
This is a highly debated topic among health-care providers and a challenging aspect of practicing remote care. The rules differ from state to state. Doctors, unlike lawyers and other professionals, have never received reimbursement for any contact between the patient and doctor that is not face-to-face, including e-mails, text, or phone discussions. Some direct-to-consumer programs have patients enrolled for a small fee per consultation. A few large health-insurance plans have accepted companies like Teladoc as a covered entity. Medicare and Medicaid have recently engaged in reimbursement for telemedicine services and cover a few specific consultations. As evidence for cost effectiveness accumulates, there is a high likelihood of more services being paid for and fewer restrictions in the near future. Other insurance plans historically follow Medicare guidelines and may do the same.

The debate continues about what is safe in telemedicine and what is not. Several cases against telehealth groups are pending in courts and awaiting final decisions. However, recent regulatory changes indicate a victory for telemedicine in general. California state has removed the seventy-two-hour limit for writing prescriptions for telemedicine patients. The Texas Medical Board has shown some leniency in approving telemedicine consults but is still restrictive. As Jonathan Linkous, CEO of ATA, wrote to the Texas board, medical practitioners have been using telemedicine since the discovery of the telephone in 1876 to treat their patients and order prescriptions. Weekend and night coverage by partners in a group practice has been an accepted custom for ages—physicians often have to make medical decisions without a face-to-face visit or a previous relationship. The potential misuse of telemedicine is a concern for all health-care providers, and constant reevaluation is in process by physical leaders to prevent it. The bottom line is that telemedicine is set to become an integral part of health care across the world, and it is a good thing.

CHAPTER 16
THE GENETIC CODE

Adriana Lopez was twenty-one years old and a new mother to six-month-old Reyna. I first met her at the high-risk-breast-cancer-screening clinic in a safety-net public hospital. She had brought her forty-seven-year-old mother, Lucia, to follow up on a blood test that had been done two weeks earlier. Lucia was diagnosed with breast cancer three months back for which she underwent a lumpectomy and radiation treatment. As per protocol, the surgeon referred her to our screening clinic for evaluation of hereditary breast cancer since she was less than fifty years old. On her first visit, she met our genetic counselor who charted out the family pedigree and ordered a blood test for the deleterious BRCA (stands for BReast CAncer) gene mutation. Two weeks later, she came to the clinic for the results of the test. Adriana was accompanying her with her daughter in a stroller—it was a profound moment for the whole family since the result of the test would inevitably affect all three generations of women.

"I am scared, Doctor," Adriana said. "I don't want my mom to die, and I don't want to die, either. We need each other."

Breast cancer is the most common cancer in women after skin cancer and the second-most common reason for cancer deaths in the United States. The risk for the average woman has been calculated to be approximately 8–10 percent, which translates to one in every ten to twelve women. However, the risk increases tremendously in those women who inherit the BRCA1 or BRCA2 mutated gene. The BRCA gene is present in all human beings and is a tumor-suppressor gene. In its normal form, it inhibits cancers in the breast, ovary, prostate, larynx, and a few other organs. When there is a deleterious mutation of this gene, the inhibitory effect disappears, thus sharply increasing the risk and incidence of cancer in the carriers, especially breast and ovarian cancer. Having said that, genetic breast cancer resulting from BRCA mutations cause only 5–10 percent of all breast cancers whereas the rest are of a sporadic nature. Among Ashkenazi Jews, 8–10 percent of women may be carriers of BRCA1 mutation (one in forty women), the highest prevalence in any ethnic group in the world.

The protocol for testing for this mutated gene is very precise—not everyone needs to get the test done. It's a very expensive test and health-insurance companies may or may not pay for it. At the safety-net public hospital where I worked, the expense was covered by a service grant from Avon. Family history of breast and ovarian cancer, especially multiple generations, younger affected women, male breast cancer, bilateral breast cancer, and both breast and ovarian cancer in one woman in the family, are highly suggestive of hereditary-cancer syndromes, one of which is the BRCA mutation. There are likely to be other hereditary-cancer types that have not yet been discovered. The person in the family who has the breast or ovarian cancer should be tested first. Once the test is found positive, another precise protocol needs to be followed, not just for the afflicted woman but also her immediate family members, including screening daughters as well as sons. Though numbers differ in

literature, overall those who carry either of the BRCA 1/2 mutations have a 40–70 percent higher risk for breast cancer and a 10–70
percent higher risk for ovarian cancer by age seventy. Personal risk
for a BRCA mutation based on family history can be calculated using several types of statistical software and models.

Unfortunately, Lucia's test for the BRCA mutation was positive.
For her, this meant that she was at a high risk of getting breast cancer in her other breast as well as ovarian cancer. She would have
to consider either a preventive bilateral mastectomy (surgically removing both breasts) or an intensive-screening follow-up with frequent mammograms and an MRI of the breasts to catch an early
breast cancer that may be curative and save her life. She would
also need preventive removal of both ovaries in a procedure called
bilateral oophorectomy. Since there are no good evidence-based
screening tests for ovarian cancer, surgical removal is recommended if the woman has completed her family and does not plan to
have another baby. Removing the ovaries would also remove the
main source of estrogen in her body and decrease her risk further
for breast cancer. In short, surgically removing both of her breasts
was not necessary but removing both of her ovaries was absolutely
necessary to reduce her cancer risk and save her life.

I discussed all the options with Lucia and Adriana and advised
them to think about her decision, discuss it with her other family members, and return in two weeks for a follow-up clinic visit. Even though
it sounds complicated, it was actually pretty straightforward for Lucia.
One way or another, we could reduce her risk for future breast and
ovarian cancers *right away* by choosing from the options above.

On the other hand, for Adriana and her infant daughter, Reyna,
it was not so simple. They were both at risk for having inherited
the gene mutation from Lucia. This possibility was frightening for

the whole family. In their limited understanding of the situation, it meant that Adriana could die from cancer at an early age. Who will take care of her infant daughter? She was engaged to Reyna's father but not married yet. How would he react to having a fiancé at very high risk of being afflicted with different types of cancer and perhaps dying from it? Would he break up with her? She also wanted to have more children. Would she pass on the defective gene to them? The social implications of being a carrier of this gene were alarming, to put it mildly. For a young, beautiful woman who had just started her family, it could essentially mean that she would have to surgically remove both of her breasts and both of her ovaries at some point in her life as primary prevention strategies to avoid getting cancer. It was a chilling thought with physical, emotional, psychological, social, and economic consequences of an extreme nature.

The first step was to check Adriana for the BRCA mutation by doing a blood test. If it was negative, Adriana and Reyna were safe, and they would be at average risk for breast and ovarian cancer like any other American woman. They just needed to follow the current age-appropriate guidelines for breast-cancer screening (there are no screening guidelines for ovarian cancer for average-risk women) at the right time. They would no longer need to schedule visits to the high-risk-screening clinic, and their care could be handled by a primary-care physician. We would have to clearly educate Adriana that the absence of the bad gene didn't mean that they were both at no risk for breast cancer—they still had the 12 percent risk that an average American woman faces. But the risk would be sporadic in nature and not hereditary, unless it was a hereditary cancer that we have no or little knowledge about.

"You have the choice of not getting tested for the gene. It's not what I recommend, but it's an option for you. Or you could take some time to decide if you want to proceed with the test," I said to Adriana.

I had met a few patients with the BRCA genetic mutation whose children just didn't want to know if they had inherited the gene, as they felt perturbed about spending the rest of their lives in perpetual anxiety. It was a choice that I respected. Everyone has the right to make choices in life and live with the consequences. I am a strong opponent of health-care providers who practice paternalistically and try to convince their patients about making decisions a certain way because *they* think it's right. I believe it putting all the options on the table and helping patients make a decision that is best for *them* in shared decision making. I may not agree with their choice, but I absolutely respect it. Thus, I felt obliged to give Adriana the choice of not being tested and dealing with problems when they happened without the rigmarole of a surveillance protocol that she may need to follow for sixty to seventy years.

Adriana, very courageously I thought, chose to get tested.

Unfortunately, the BRCA mutation test was positive for Adriana too. This really complicated matters. So what do we do now? What are the best options for Adriana? What about little Reyna? The goals for her were the same as Lucia—to try to reduce the risk of breast and ovarian cancer as much as possible. The critical difference was her age—she was too young and had not completed her family yet. The option to remove both of her ovaries—to decrease her risk for ovarian cancer to negligible and for breast cancer substantially (by 50 percent)—was a difficult and grave decision for her. She still needed her ovaries for having more children, *and* at the age of twenty-one, she needed estrogen to avoid early menopause that would put her at life-threatening risk for cardiovascular disease, osteoporosis, dementia, and debilitating hot flashes. Her overall risk for morbidity, quality of life, and life expectancy could be affected sharply with her ovaries removed so early. But keeping them would raise her risk for ovarian cancer to up to 39 percent as compared to average women whose risk was 1.3 percent. She still had the option of choosing a bilateral mastectomy to decrease her risk for breast cancer. But she was young, and a drastic surgery like this could have an incredibly negative psychosocial impact. Instead, she could opt for intensive-surveillance screening at six-month intervals with a mammogram and an MRI for the rest of her life, starting at age twenty-five, as well as clinical breast examinations by her doctor at regular intervals. A tough set of decisions for the patient as well as the doctor.

In recent times, many celebrities have been diagnosed with the BRCA gene mutation with or without breast and ovarian cancer. For health-care providers like us it has been a sort of boon to have this problem receive attention from the medical community as well as the media since it spreads awareness in the public. The star who got the most media attention was Angelina Jolie. There were others like Guiliana Rancic and Cristina Applegate, both of whom had early breast cancer in their thirties and were found to have the mutated gene. All three chose a bilateral mastectomy. Eventually they will need their ovaries removed too—that is, once they have completed their families. Specialists strongly recommend that ovaries be removed by age forty to prevent ovarian cancer. Pierce Brosnan's daughter died at the age of thirty-eight from ovarian cancer. Her mother Cassandra Harris, Brosnan's first wife, also died of ovarian cancer at an early age, and it was recommended that her daughter undergo surgical removal of both of her ovaries, though it is not public knowledge if they carried the BRCA mutation. She refused the surgery and was afflicted by the cancer, which unfortunately resulted in her demise, leaving behind two children. This conflict is quite common among persons with the mutated gene. In our clinic, we have several patients who refuse the removal of their ovaries. Why go through a surgery when there are no symptoms, and it's not bothering them? The physiological complexity of the sequence of events is often confusing for patients to completely comprehend. Sometimes it requires repeated visits to the specialist for a reiteration of the rationale behind the surgery. Until they decide to undergo surgery, a less-than-adequate regimen of pelvic ultrasound and testing for a tumor marker for ovarian cancer are recommended—neither is a good screening test, but together they are better than nothing.

Angelina Jolie, unlike the others, was not diagnosed with breast cancer. Her mother died of ovarian cancer at an early age as did her maternal grandmother. This family history was enough to test her for the deleterious BRCA gene mutation, which was positive. She was given all the options above and chose to undergo a double mastectomy and more recently, removal of both of her ovaries.

This is a very courageous decision by any standards. It makes it even more so, considering that her career in showbiz is largely based on outward appearances in general and specifically for her, a sex symbol from Hollywood. The double mastectomy is a very painful surgery that could take weeks and months to recover from. Women often go home with drains hanging from their chest to prevent any collection of oozing fluid at the surgical site that could get infected, an arduous and challenging situation to be confronted with on a daily basis. Frequent follow-up office visits for a tissue "expander implant" are needed—a temporary device filled with a small amount of saline that is placed under the chest wall, and expanded every one to three weeks with an injection of approximately 50 ml of saline. The purpose is to gradually create a space for the actual implant in a second reconstructive surgery for women who choose that option. This whole process is very grueling, anxiety provoking, uncomfortable, and tiring. Cosmetically, what it does to a woman's body and mind is unfathomable for the untrained layperson and incredibly difficult to describe in mere words for me. Most women with the BRCA mutation in our clinic, and probably overall, thus choose intensive surveillance over a double mastectomy, even though the procedure could reduce the risk for cancer to under 5 percent. Jolie's story has inevitably given many women the nerve to make choices for themselves that they might not have made before knowing about her experience.

Certainly more women are opting for a double mastectomy as their choice of treatment if they are carriers of the BRCA gene. However, Adriana decided not to get either a double mastectomy or oophorectomy. Instead, she opted for frequent clinical breast examinations and intensive screening starting at age twenty-five with alternate mammogram and breast MRI every six months. She wanted to try to have one more child as soon as possible. Until then, a pelvic ultrasound to evaluate her ovaries and tumor-marker blood tests for ovarian cancer were requested at regular intervals—though these were not ideal screening tests for ovarian cancer, something was better than nothing. The ultimate goal was to be able to catch a cancer really early and provide curative treatment. Later in her life, she could decide if she wanted to continue screening for breast cancer or get a double mastectomy. Once she completed her family, she would be ready for the surgical removal of both of her ovaries. Clearly, she would need a multidisciplinary team of specialists and superspecialists, genetic counselors, nurses, and navigating staff for the rest of her life. Her daughter, Reyna, and other children could decide to get genetic testing when they attained adulthood and became capable of grasping the intricacies of the treatment options to choose the best for themselves.

One of the controversies surrounding the BRCA1 and BRCA2 genes has been their patenting by Myriad Genetics, the laboratory that held a monopoly on testing for the gene mutation for years. Several lawsuits were filed against them, decrying the ethics and moral principle of patenting a human gene. The Supreme Court ruled that these patents were invalid, thus ending Myriad's monopoly in gene testing. How can anyone patent naturally occurring DNA? Technically then, anyone could patent any part of the body! It was even suggested that Angelina Jolie had timed her surgery and the news release to coincide with the Supreme Court judgment, that she was in cahoots with Myriad, and there was a pact of some sort between them, all intended to milk the situation for money and other secondary gain. It seemed really far-fetched to me at many different levels. For one thing, you would have to be very hardcore and indestructible to find out that you are at very high risk of dying from cancer, undergo one of the toughest surgeries that a woman can experience, have six young children who could become motherless, and at the same time plan a *business venture* with a commercial partner to gain from your medical problems! It's possible that Jolie was that resilient. Personally, I doubt it. The Supreme Court verdict silenced the buzz and her critics, as it was against Myriad. There was no money to be made. Since then, other companies have started offering the gene testing at a lower price than Myriad, instigating more litigation and legal wrangling.

All this over a piece of my DNA!

CHAPTER 17

UNRAVELING A FOOD MYSTERY

About half a dozen years ago, I started noticing certain non-specific symptoms that were beginning to affect my quality of life. I had steady painless bloating of the abdomen that made me look pregnant by the end of the day and feel rather uncomfortable. This mysterious abdominal distension was very unnerving—it was as if someone was intentionally pumping tiny amounts of air into my stomach all day, like inflating a basketball. I had trouble with my clothes not fitting well in the evening. People asked me if I was pregnant. I could even see the potbelly in pictures.

Other symptoms also appeared insidiously like fatigue, irritability, gurgling, and a vague abdominal discomfort. Some days I had swelling of my face, fingers, and feet, and I could not get my wedding ring off my finger. Other days it would slip out easily. Sometimes my face looked so swollen that my eyelids were practically slits. People around me noticed it. A close friend once asked me why my face "looked so big." Against my best instincts, I started using over-the-counter laxatives. I felt intense relief within a few hours but it did not answer any questions. I was oddly fearful to see a gastroenterologist, as I knew that the doctor would recommend a colonoscopy, and I was not excited to get one.

Over the next few years, I struggled every day. Suddenly one day it dawned on me like an epiphany—could gluten be the problem?

My diet was replete with bread as the main source of grains. Trips to the grocery store always included several types of "designer bread." To test my hypothesis, I went on a gluten-free diet. There was a dramatic resolution of all the symptoms. I reintroduced a gluten challenge to prove a temporal relation. All the symptoms reappeared within hours, and they persisted for several days, suggesting the possibility of gluten intolerance. Changing my diet has been difficult but incredibly helpful. Interestingly, when I think of my childhood, I remember my younger sister getting abdominal cramps from highly processed wheat flour. That was more than forty years ago. She learned to stay away from certain types of foods that used the dough from processed wheat. Whole wheat never caused her any problems. Her daughter, now fourteen, has also had several episodes of acute abdominal symptoms with restaurant pizzas and similar foods, though she tolerates whole wheat well. Indeed gluten-related disorders have existed for a long time.

The literature is replete with studies and reviews about gluten enteropathy, a heterogeneous group of disorders that includes gluten intolerance, gluten sensitivity, gluten allergy, and celiac disease, all occurring because of the effect of gluten on the intestinal system. The latest nomenclature (see below) describes a wide spectrum of gluten-related disorders (GRD), the prevalence of which has been on the rise for several reasons, particularly the increasing use of wheat instead of other grains like rice (as in the Mediterranean diet) and the supposed higher content of gluten in wheat these days as compared to old times. The wheat eaten ten thousand years ago was a lot different in gluten content and quality from the current variety. Technology has been blamed for the higher gluten content in current wheat. Conversely, studies have been done that disprove this theory that wheat breeding has disproportionately increased gluten content over the years, thus contributing to a higher prevalence of GRD. Additionally, there have been claims that the overuse of antibiotics and excessive hygienic practices may also lead to GRD.

The role of genetically modified foods in aggravating GRD is controversial. Some scientists and green groups allege that genetic engineering can cause gluten sensitivity in two ways—altering the protective gut bacteria and directly damaging the intestinal cells that cause permeability, or leakiness. Glyphosate, an active but toxic ingredient of a weed killer to which genetically modified crops are engineered to be resistant, has been blamed for causing such damage. However, no scientific evidence-based studies have been done to prove or disprove this theory. Furthermore, genetically engineered wheat is yet to be produced commercially in the United States.

"Gluten-free" is a term that is much bandied about. In fact, those in high-society circles have controversially identified it as just a fad. Restaurants serve gluten-free foods and grocery stores often have an entire section for gluten-free products, which are more expensive than regular products. Cynics have often described this as more of a trend that is considered "hip" and "cool" and remain skeptical about the existence of a real disorder.

So what is gluten?

Gluten is a protein composite that acts as glue (thus the name) to help the dough rise and keep the shape of the food. This widely consumed component of food is present in wheat, rye, oat, barley, spelt, triticale, and kamut. It may be native to the food itself or an additive intended to alter the characteristics of the product. Since wheat provides half the calories in food for the entire world, gluten-enriched food is ubiquitously available and eaten extensively. The higher the gluten content, the more the elasticity of the food. The chewiness of bagels, garlic breads, and pizzas is because of high gluten content, which changes the texture of bread. It may even be present in cosmetics and hair products. The Western food market generally has higher gluten content in its items than the developing world, partly because of the cost of adding gluten.

Historically, gluten was considered to play a causal role in celiac disease, a relatively serious disorder that was thought to be limited to Europe and of infrequent occurrence. Thus, it received sparse attention from the medical world. Celiac disease is an extreme form of gluten sensitivity that spurs a strong immunological reaction in the body, causing an array of symptomatology that may be life threatening. There is an inflammation of the lining of the intestines, and tests may reveal the presence of immune markers in the blood. Symptoms include diarrhea, intestinal bloating, gas, fatigue, anemia, and weight loss. Some patients get joint pain and migraine headaches. Eventually, if gluten is not withheld in the diet, the lining of the intestines is destroyed to the point that nutrients are not absorbed adequately from the gut, leading to a host of complications. This autoimmune disease can be present from birth or may be acquired as we grow older. In fact, Dr. Alessio Fasano from the Center for Celiac Disease Research at the University of Maryland once said in a statement, "We can never be too old to get celiac disease." The only treatment available for celiac disease is a gluten-free diet. A portion of patients may suffer life-threatening symptoms, even with trace quantities of gluten.

However, since the 1970s, the incidence of celiac disease in the United States has doubled every fifteen years that has garnered the attention of health-care providers and researchers. According to the National Institutes of Health, it is now estimated that one in one hundred forty-one people suffers from celiac disease in the country. Recently, scientists have also recognized another group of disorders called nonceliac gluten sensitivity. Patients with such intolerance have symptoms of celiac disease but because of the lack of intestinal inflammation, there is no ongoing or residual damage to the intestines. The standard immunological blood tests done for celiac disease are negative in these patients. Such patients benefit from consuming gluten-free foods to varying degrees but are not at risk for life-threatening complications with a gluten load. Science is still unclear about the exact sequence of events that occur with gluten sensitivity.

In 2011, experts met in London to outline the best nomenclature for GRD. According to them, it encompasses three different conditions: (a) autoimmune disorders—celiac disease, dermatitis herpetiformis (a skin condition), and gluten ataxia (a neurological condition); (b) allergic disorder—wheat allergy; and (c) nonallergic, nonautoimmune disorder—gluten sensitivity. Patients with wheat allergy get asthma-like respiratory symptoms (also known as baker's asthma), a skin rash, as well as intestinal symptoms. A skin allergy test is diagnostic and widely available. I suspect I fall into the last category, as do a large number of people who follow a gluten-free diet with relief of their symptoms but no objective evidence of gluten intolerance biochemically or histologically. This diagnosis is based on clinical symptoms only and is one of exclusion of other types of GRD.

How do people react differently to gluten? What determines whether one will get celiac disease or simple intolerance? To answer these questions it is important to understand the structure of gluten in wheat. It is essentially composed of two major proteins—glutenin and gliadin. Gliadin has several different epitopes, and the reaction to a certain epitope determines what type of GRD will be manifested. For example, an immunological reaction to alpha-gliadin is the pathological process inherent to celiac disease. Once in the gut, an enzyme called transglutaminase, which is also of different types, then digests gluten. Antibodies to these also occur in GRD as part of the pathological process. However, a specific reaction to type 2 transglutaminase occurs in celiac disease. Wheat and other grains also contain other types of proteins. People can react to any of these proteins or their subtypes and manifest symptoms similar to celiac disease. The protein fraction that induces their systemic reaction determines the type of GRD they manifest. However, it is critical to understand that current investigative technology can detect only those antibodies, which cause celiac disease as described above. This indicates that you may have negative tests for celiac disease but still have a diagnosis of gluten intolerance or sensitivity. In the future, it may be possible to detect reactions to all different epitopes and subtypes that will help in the correct diagnosis and treatment of nonceliac gluten intolerance.

It has also been noted that some people with no gluten intolerance choose to go gluten free without a medical necessity, justifying it as a healthier choice. Gluten has been blamed for other disorders like schizophrenia, autism, attention-deficit hyperactivity disorder, irritable bowel syndrome, and multiple sclerosis, though there is no scientific evidence of this relationship. Anecdotes of clinical improvement in these conditions with a gluten-free diet are very common but not proven by research.

It is entirely possible that unidentified genes may predispose us to gluten sensitivity. In some studies, it has been claimed that innovators, thinkers, and achievers of modern times are more likely to buy gluten-free products! Oh well, I don't mind any of these adjectives for myself. Naysayers against a gluten-free diet have expressed their concern that a gluten-free diet may strip us of nutrients like vitamin B and folic acid, as well as fiber, all of which are essential components of a balanced diet. An abnormal alteration of gut bacteria can weaken the immune system. At times, it may just be a ploy to mask an eating disorder or to lose weight in a socially acceptable manner. One of my close friends once snidely remarked that it was a convenient way to avoid carbohydrates, hinting that losing weight was my main objective. The food industry, already ostracized for brainwashing and fooling the public, has been accused of rushing in to take advantage of a foolproof business opportunity. Add to this, the cost and inconvenience, and we have a conspiracy theory!

The Food and Drug Administration announced in 2013 that "in order to use the term 'gluten-free,' 'no gluten,' 'free of gluten,' and 'without gluten' on its label, a food must meet all the requirements of the definition, including that the food must contain less than twenty parts per million of gluten." Approximately 4 percent of American adults buy gluten-free products, though less than one-fifth may have been diagnosed with a gluten-related disorder. Gluten-free foods, therefore, now have sales of more than $2.6 billion annually in the Unites States, higher than foods for a fat-free diet or a low-carbohydrate diet. The *New York Times* projected that by 2016 the sales will top $15 billion. The persistent upward trend, as compared to more of a bell curve for other fad diets, could be because of the wider profit margins and dissimilar dynamics of the gluten-free food market.

One of my patients with GRD once showed me a pack of "gluten cutters" in the form of capsules that she uses when she eats gluten-loaded foods. She claimed that these enzyme-laden capsules really helped her digest these foods better and were available at general stores like Walgreens. Inspired by her, I bought a pack of gluten-cutter capsules and used them after eating a high-gluten meal. I also added expensive probiotics to my regimen to promote digestion. The only change that I have experienced with these remedies is a biopsy of my wallet. Staying away from glutinous foods is the single remedy that has really helped me with my symptoms. I tried eating gluten-free foods but gagged at the frightfully unappetizing flavors. Pizza tasted like fine sand, and sliced bread was more like slabs of solidified powder. On an international flight, I once ordered gluten-free meals and was handed a plate with a dry sandwich consisting of two desiccated pieces of rice toast with cheese and a few veggies inside. The steward gave me a sympathetic glance and said, "It's not much, I see." I remained hungry throughout the ten-hour flight and swore off any special meal requests for life. Thank God for trail mix!

A fad diet? Maybe so. But I am never going to go back to eating unrestricted breads like before. I suspect millions of Americans will agree with me.

CHAPTER 18

AN ODE TO COUNTY

Heaven knows we need never be ashamed of our tears, for they are rain upon the blinding dust of earth, overlying our hard hearts. I was better after I had cried, than before—more sorry, more aware of my own ingratitude, more gentle.

—Charles Dickens, *Great Expectations*

No book written by me would be complete without a heartfelt account of my stint at Cook County Hospital in Chicago, fondly known simply as County. Yes, there were tears. At times, I felt better after I had cried; at other times I did not. I was always more sorry and more aware of my ingratitude. I saw more of what was already there to be seen, but remained unseen. I heard in the silence, a resonance that was often drowned in the thuds and hums and jingles of daily life. I felt it every now and then, that touch, sometimes a caress, sometimes a graze, a scratch, a bruise, a wound, a deep gash.

"We are all wounded, including you," said a young girl I met recently, the daughter of a sex worker in Mumbai, to an audience of affluent Indians who had come to watch a play. It made so much sense. Everyone has a story. And everyone thinks that his or her story is the most compelling. Until you encounter another one that leaves you dazed. Or several stories, each more riveting than the last, that swamp you in an overwhelming motley of sensations— grief, despair, anguish, and torment, alongside hope, faith, courage, joy, and sometimes delight.

My son asked me why I wanted to dedicate the last chapter of my book to County. The reason is not complicated. County not only shaped who I am as a health-care provider but also changed me as a person. It helped me define success for myself—the ability to make a difference in the lives of other people. At County I saw a side of the country that only a handful of Americans get to see, the dirty side that remains muted and hushed. I saw hunger, deprivation, injustice, poverty, prejudice, discrimination, and a disparity not unlike developing countries in Africa and Asia. But within that lumbering beast was an incredible island of hope and comfort that sustained the lives of countless individuals from across the world, without heed to color, race, ethnicity, language, gender, legal status, health insurance, or income—just being human was enough.

Cook County Hospital is the third-largest public hospital in the United States after New York and Los Angeles county hospitals, a safety-net institution that caters predominantly to the vulnerable population of Chicago. A hospital is composed of a set of different elements—medical, administrative, research, volunteer, social, rehabilitative, and so on. But the core component that drives the success of a hospital is the medical team led by doctors. Dr. Robert Weinstein, past chairperson of the department of medicine, and a pioneer in academia, frequently said,

"There are two kinds of physicians: those who *work* at County and those who *want* to work at County." Indeed, the physicians who work at County choose to do so out of a sense of service for the vulnerable population, unparalleled in the history of health care in the United States. This last chapter is my token of gratitude to them for teaching me what my life should be about and what it means to make a difference selflessly in the lives of others.

My journey with County began when I did not even understand the meaning of a "safety-net" hospital or the "vulnerable" population. After completing my residency, I became immersed in private practice in an affluent neighborhood in Chicago. It was a difficult five years for me. Medical malpractice litigations were sprouting every day, and Illinois was one of the worst hit. Health-policy reform was a touchy subject. Medicare regulations were rigid, and physician reimbursement was declining rapidly. I found my work tedious and unrewarding. But the two factors that bothered me the most were the lack of time or space for academic and scholarly activities, and the absence of a cohesive health-care system for the poor and underprivileged. County provided an answer to both.

I felt incredibly excited when I started working there as a fellow in preventive medicine. The buzzing, chaotic pace meant there was never a dull moment. The ethnic diversity was comforting and reassuring. I knew I was in the right place. Later on, my mentor would confide in me how he could tell immediately that I was a good fit for County. Every day was a new experience. I felt inspired by the scholars, residents, students, nurses, and social workers and their absolute commitment to making things happen for the patients. Going beyond the call of duty was the norm. For none more so than the attending physicians who stunned me by their devotion to the mission statement of County—"to deliver integrated health services with dignity and respect regardless of a patient's ability to pay." I understood honestly what it meant to be true advocates for your patients, to fight the system to serve them, how compassion can touch lives beyond the tangible, why small things matter the most—like a hug, a smile, a high five, a wave—and that nothing counts more in medicine than the human touch.

Where else would you find the associate director of the internal medicine residency program standing in line at the outpatient pharmacy with a patient's prescription, waiting with a number to be called to collect the medicines? I normally avoided crossing the first-floor pharmacy area to reach my clinic. It was always overcrowded with patients, and I felt depressed, knowing that some of them had been waiting for hours for their medications to be ready for pickup. My colleague must have stood there a long time.

Year after year, another colleague of mine in the division of general internal medicine chose a four-week inpatient call rotation in the summer. I asked her why she did it. Summer was an unpopular period to purposely choose an inpatient service, as it was vacation time for school kids. We could choose a two-week call instead of four weeks, if at all. It gives my partners who have children a break, she said. She was single and had no children of her own. How thoughtful. The same thoughtfulness was evident in her care for patients.

A few years ago, Dr. Gordon Schiff, a very senior clinician from County who moved to Boston to work at Harvard University, was reprimanded by the Brigham and Women's Hospital. He had given a patient thirty dollars on a Friday evening to buy medicines for an acute problem that her health-insurance company refused to discuss or pay for. This incident spurred an intense discussion on boundaries between patients and their health-care providers. Are so-called unwritten professional boundaries more critical to the central core of practicing medicine than being kind? Would most of my County colleagues have done the same? The answer is yes, because they care for the patient as a whole. What good was an office visit, a consultation, and a three-page documentation by the physician if the patient does not have the means to get treatment? How often do we find ourselves in this situation? Every prescribed medication had a preset copay of four dollars at the County pharmacy, for a maximum of twenty dollars per person. Most patients were on several life-saving, long-term medications and could not afford the copays. It was an open secret that patients got help from their providers in many different but ordinary ways, acts worthy of condemnation in the medical community as getting too close for comfort and crossing boundaries that were never meant to be crossed to preserve the professional relationships. "Secretly committing simple acts of kindness"—this was how Dr. Schiff described it. To punish a highly esteemed physician for a simple act of kindness seems extreme, as if it was a crime, one that my County colleagues were never shy of committing. What grievous harm could giving a patient thirty dollars to buy medications possibly do? He went on to describe how the best antidote to physician burnout is to strive for an eloquent meaningful relationship with our patients in which we don't just solve "problems" but indulge in compassionate, empathetic care that makes being a physician highly rewarding. It's not as complex to understand as quantum physics or rocket science—we choose to be doctors for a reason, and that reason is simple. We want to help people. Not just write prescriptions but actually follow ordinary humanitarian principles and provide care and comfort. Isn't it cruel to punish us for being kind?

My mentor and guide at County, now retired, was someone who had never had a job at another hospital in his entire life after medical school. He completed his residency and continued as an attending physician at County until the day he retired. When I first started working there, I was told as an aside from another senior physician that "he is considered God at County." I felt puzzled, and I didn't quite understand what she meant until I had worked with him for a while. Indeed, he was godlike. I learned from him that eye contact with the patient and body language were the most critical aspects of the office visit. I watched him turn away from the computer, pull his chair close to the patient, look directly at them, and bend forward, giving his whole attention to listen. He hardly spoke and never interrupted. Listen more, talk less. Not so easy for physicians—a study clearly showed that physicians wait for only twenty-three seconds before interrupting their patient at the start of a visit. Patient satisfaction is much higher when there is an attentive but mostly silent physician. This lesson has made me a better person, not just at work but also in my personal life. It is a powerful message to young doctors, especially since laws for "meaningful use" of electronic medical records compel health-care providers to connect deeply with the inanimate computer but only cursorily with the animate patient.

One day, a couple of years into working at County, I was walking toward the elevator to go up to my academic office for lunch. The swipe machine was right outside the double doors leading to the atrium where the elevators were, and I took the opportunity to swipe my identity card as proof of my daily attendance. As I turned around, the double doors opened, and I saw a huge cart with multiple large cartons on it being wheeled out in the opposite direction. I could not see who was pushing the cart, since the boxes were piled high on top of one another. I stepped closer to hold one of the doors open and was amazed to see the program director of the internal medicine residency program, a slender, petite woman, pushing it all by herself! I exclaimed in surprise and asked her if she needed help. The load seemed humongous for her. As always, she smiled elegantly and said she was OK. She had lugged the cart down all the way from the fifteenth floor of one building to cross over to the hospital to take it several floors higher. I could tell this wasn't the first time she had done this. She could have had the transporters do this for her or even requested one of the residents, or the janitors, or anyone else. It was not her job to haul cargo. As the director of one of the biggest residency programs in the country, she had her work cut out for her. But she led by example—going beyond the call of duty. No task was too small, no errand menial. Embedded in our roles at County was the unsaid belief that if we try hard enough we can do it, whatever it was that we wanted to. I heard of legendary past physicians who brought a mop and cleaning spray to the general-medicine clinic in the Fantus building, an old, somewhat dilapidated four-story structure that was not very clean. Others brought flowers to cheer up the nurses and medical assistants.

A younger colleague who had to move to another state invited some of her patients for lunch at the clinic prior to leaving. I was surprised, as I had never heard of doctors doing that. Any farewell get-together was usually among the caregivers. Many doctors attended weddings and birthdays in the homes of patients. All of us got gifts from our patients, including food, clothing, jewelry, and so on. This may seem usual at other medical practices but remember, our patients often had no money to buy their medicines. Yet they found ways to show the doctors their gratitude. We often asked them, especially those who lived far away or had health insurance, why they continued their care at County when they could choose another institution. The wait was terrible, it was overcrowded, the system had many problems, and the pharmacy was overstretched. The answer was always the same—we love the doctors; they are the best in the world.

And the best of the best? The palliative-care team was an exceptionally dedicated and awe-inspiring crew of providers who strived relentlessly to serve the weakest and most fragile of the vulnerable patients—those with terminal cancers or serious illnesses. For them, there was the clinical aspect of prescribing medications for comfort care, improving the quality of life of patients and their families, and coordinating care for transition from hospital to nursing home to home and often back to the hospital, in a circle that could frequently be vicious and incessant. And then there was the ethical and moral piece that was inherent to their job description. "Home" often meant another country like Mexico, Poland, Guatemala, or Panama, and writing letters to foreign embassies for patients or their families to coordinate care was an integral part of their daily routine. Many terminally ill patients wanted nothing more than to die in their country of birth. The US consulates in many of these countries knew our palliative care team well; any letter from them with recommendations was taken seriously and acted upon immediately. Maybe a family member needed a visa; maybe there was a concern that needed to be addressed on the patient's flight back home; maybe travel tickets needed an adjustment because of an unforeseen emergency. It all was taken care of, regardless of time and resources.

I miss working at County. It's an ache that never goes away. I miss my patients the most. Moving away was hard, but the most difficult part was the conversation I had with each one of them to bid good-bye. There were tears, sometimes loud sobbing, occasionally anger, but mostly disappointment. A few took the news stoically. I felt emotionally exhausted. We promised to keep in touch, knowing well that it would probably not happen, that we would never meet again. A handful said they would no longer seek care at County, as they could not conceive changing physicians. My biggest concern was the possible attrition and loss of follow-up that comes with a change in health-care providers. I made sure that most of them had follow-up appointments with other primary-care physicians.

A few weeks ago, I received a call from a funeral home in Chicago. They wanted me to sign the death certificate of one of my patients. My initial reaction was utter shock—she was too young to die even though she had a very complex medical history. The last time I had seen her was a year and a half ago. Apparently, she never went back to see my replacement physician. Maybe she sought care elsewhere; there was no way to know. It was heartbreaking to think of all the times we had met, chatted about this and that, confided in each other about our lives' turns, hugged after the visit, and bid that last farewell with a promise that she would watch her health closely. Even though the mind knows that I may never meet any of my County patients again, the heart holds a flicker of hope that it may happen. And if it did, we would shout in joyous wonder when our eyes met, embrace in a bear hug, and catch up on all that we missed! Sadly, that flicker was forever snuffed out for this person.

But *this* was County—the patient-physician bond was unlike any other. It was one big dysfunctional family that worked well in one dimension and was incredibly worn out in another. The cracks and fissures were visible for all to see, but that bond was cement that kept it from falling apart. We reveled in it. There was an indescribable exuberance about County that was intangible but also infinite—a powerful and heady mix of optimism and confidence, an audacious anticipation of hope and courage amid a tumultuous groundswell of goodwill that resonated through foyers and antechambers and vestibules of the maze that was Cook County Hospital, a.k.a John H. Stroger Jr. Hospital of Cook County. The nameless County physician was the maze runner, gliding in and out of those cracks and fissures, healing and curing, soothing and easing, a stroke here and a caress there, a whisper of promise, a soft reassurance, a boundless cheer, that everything would be OK, that no hurdle was high enough, and in the end we will win. Even hundreds of miles away I can feel it, sense it, perceive it—an overpowering deluge of memories forever embedded in my spirit that besieges me enchantingly.

Until all that I am left with are waves of nostalgia, a longing of the soul, and the sounds of a stethoscope.

ACKNOWLEDGEMENTS

This book was written at a time when almost everyone in my life that I loved was sick. In retrospect, it was a blessing in disguise. It forced me to rearrange my priorities and led me to the life I lead now, a much happier one. I am always grateful for that.

I want to thank all those who I consider mentors and role models in my career, without whom neither would I have a meaningful career, nor this book: Dr. David Goldberg, who taught me everything about research methods and from whom I understood what compassion really means; Dr. Catherine Deamant, who inspired me endlessly with her dedication to the terminally ill; Dr. Krishna Das, who taught me the nuts and bolts of patient safety; Dr. Rudolf Kumapley, from whom I learned the nuances of teaching; Dr. Pamela Ganshow, who taught me everything about women's health; and all my colleagues, residents, and students I have ever worked with – I learned something from each one.

I want to thank my husband, son, parents, and niece for helping me write this book with their constant support and encouragement.

And last but not the least – my patients. You are, and will always be, my muse. Without you, all I have is nothingness.